—TOM BLACKMAN—

TARGET LEAN

Published by Goldcrest Books International Ltd
www.goldcrestbooks.com
publish@goldcrestbooks.com

ISBN: 978-1-911505-78-5
eISBN: 978-1-911505-79-2

To my daughter Ellie.

I stole and ate her Easter eggs in 2010, when she was 8 years old, while dieting for a show. That was the turning point for me to learn and ultimately to teach a new way of eating for a leaner body.

CONTENTS

FOREWORD

Five years ago, I welcomed in our new 2015 cohort of graduate students to what was going to be the start of a very exciting but steep learning journey in sport and exercise nutrition. I recall vividly the lecture room being packed full of eager students from various corners of the world, who were in London specifically for our regular quarterly "taught weekend' sessions. They would be exposed to a truly world-class line-up of top academics (often the ones conducting and publishing the actual research being studied) and elite practitioners (typically working with Olympic squads, world champion boxers, national teams, professional premier-league rugby and football teams etc). These sessions supplemented the 1200 hours of online study and additional lectures on advanced level exercise physiology and nutrition science that comprise just some of the challenging elements of the course that they were to undertake. Amongst the 40 or so students attending, consisting primarily of those with undergraduate degrees in sport science, nutrition and dietetics, were 2 very large (or more accurately "hulk" like) men in the front-row in tight t-shirts and bulging biceps, along with a carefully arranged assortment of protein bars, monster energy drinks and assorted tubs of pre-prepared calorie-controlled high-protein meals in Tupperware. To say they were not typical of the rest of the students would be an understatement! Like many bodybuilders and physique competitors, these big guys were extraordinarily hungry all the time – and not just for food but also for knowledge to help them and their clients achieve optimal results through their physical training and dietary endeavours.

One of these hulks was Tom Blackman. Right from that very first day, Tom's voracious thirst for knowledge was evidenced in everything he did on the course, always sitting in the front row and asking the professors well thought out questions in a genuine attempt to understand the highly complex science being presented. Over the course of the next several years through sheer hard work and dedication to his studies, Tom demonstrated mastery of the subject, with an impressive evolution of this hulk into a distinction grade graduate of the program. No mean feat!

In *Target Lean*, Tom evidences his mastery of nutrition and behaviour change. This book is a valuable tool to the reader, because it achieves one especially significant and yet very rare accomplishment which is that it manages to bridge the gap between evidence-based science and "real world" application. It may surprise you to know that there is often a big difference between knowing (i.e. the science) and doing (i.e. successfully applying it to achieve a desired result).

As an elite practitioner Tom has put in years of study as well as many years' experience applying the science to practice, successfully, on not only himself but also on hundreds of clients at the highest level. In order to do this he needed to spend many hundreds of hours learning the complex science and acquire the critical thinking skills that are required to be able to differentiate the quality from flawed information that exists in abundance and that is promulgated on social media and other channels by self-proclaimed "nutrition experts", and then develop ways in which to guide and support its application into everyday life.

In this book, therefore, Tom has sourced and translated the relevant high quality information into an easy to read and practical to apply format that you the reader can realistically and effectively benefit from. Tom has done the hard work and genuinely cares about you and your goals to be healthy and lean. In this book I am confident that you can trust in his advice and undertake this exciting and long-lasting journey with his assistance on what will be a thoroughly rewarding journey toward a healthier and leaner you!

Dr Laurent Bannock DProf MSc RNutr SENr
Founder and Director,
The Institute of Performance Nutrition
London, UK

1. INTRODUCTION

It's 2004 and I'm backstage at the UK Bodybuilding Finals; back then it was called the EFBB, the English Federation of Bodybuilders. It was my first year competing at this event after qualifying at the South Coast Championship, in second place.

I was in good spirits going into the show, and as everyone stood backstage, tanned and oiled up and in their pants, I looked around and knew that I probably wasn't going to win, or be placed that year, as there were so many other very good bodybuilders with much more experience than me.

I looked good, of course. I'd been dieting for over sixteen weeks to get to that point and I was definitely in decent shape, just not the highest quality needed for a British finals placing, so I decided to ask a few of the other guys what they did on their diets.

"I do Keto," said one.

"High carbs for me," said another.

"Low carbs then high fats on rotation," was a third response.

At this point in my life I didn't have any real nutrition education; I'd got into shape by basically just starving myself of carbohydrates and eating chicken and broccoli every day coupled with a few hours of cardio chucked in for good measure.

I was unaware of any of the research into nutrition, so I and many of my co-competitors relied on secrets handed down from former bodybuilders, which we then applied to our own diets and training schedules to get to where we needed to be.

If the diet wasn't working, we just dropped off more carbs, or did more cardio, or took more fat-burning supplements. It's the reality of the sport I was involved in; extreme fat loss called for extreme measures.

Of course, this left us in a bit of a dark place generally. Bodybuilders often have a reputation for being moody and grumpy, a bit snappy and mentally slow from the carb depletion, and we would never go anywhere without our Tupperware of smelly chicken or white fish and steamed vegetables. I was *not* the exception to this rule.

We were great fun at parties, mostly because we were never there to spoil it for others as we became hermits and recluses, focussing on our five minutes on stage to win the trophy.

Sometimes all this worked, and we won.

A lot of the time though, it didn't, and we failed to hit our mark. That was to be the order of the day for me. I wasn't as 'shredded' – a bodybuilding term for low body fat – as the other guys, and not as big, so I placed dead-last. I was not happy and still no wiser as to how I could improve for the next show. I was incredibly frustrated at my failure and blamed myself for the mess up.

"I wasn't hard enough on myself or my diet."

"I didn't do enough cardio."

"I should have cut carbs out like that other guy that won, he looked awesome."

This completed the cycle of events that I've come to know as the three core-influencing factors that inflict pressure and prevent a person reaching the fat-loss targets they have.

Whether you're a bodybuilder looking to get ripped for a show, or a new mum looking to shift the baby weight, these factors will apply to you.

The core factors are, in essence, barriers to your success. They create problems for you, and interfere in your life with the effect of limiting your fat-burning progress. More on these in a minute.

2. THE RECKONING

After that competition where I totally bombed out, I decided that I would learn everything I could about nutrition. Originally, it was so I could be a better bodybuilder and win more shows without having a near-death experience. Later on it became a career that I loved, and still do today.

When I say 'near-death experience' I am not joking. That day I was so dehydrated that I could only open doors by leaning into them. I had no strength and didn't encapsulate the muscular, strong appearance I outwardly portrayed. This is a common occurrence in many physique competitions and people have ended up in hospital due to pushing the boundaries of their health to look good. Sadly, this is also true of many people trying to lose body fat, and something I have made it my goal to eradicate.

At this time, like many athletes, I had a normal office job to pay the bills. Bodybuilding doesn't pay the bills, it creates them, lots of them. The amount of food and supplements

I would get through each week was staggering. I'd also spend numerous hours in the gym, crafting and shaping the physique that I wanted to present on stage.

I didn't really care about my job – it was in a small local council and the work was boring. It meant that I could live the life of a bodybuilder and focus everything on being the best I could be on stage. As boring as the work was, it was also very easy. I could do a day's work in a few hours, which left me a lot of time to plan the opening of my own gym.

After a nine-month battle with the local governing council of the area, and a lot of underhand tactics by the planning officer, I managed to secure planning permission for my gym. You can read more about the many issues and obstacles the council threw at me on my gym's website: www.mofgym.co.uk

What this meant was that I now owned my own gym and I could finally pursue an additional career in nutrition. This was in 2010 and six years after my initial decision to learn more about nutrition.

I'd been working with a few people as a side hustle, writing diet plans for them to help with their own nutrition, to earn a bit of extra cash. I'd also been reading everything I could about nutrition from magazines and websites. At this point I wasn't aware of the huge amount of research data that was freely available on PubMed, and as a result a lot of the information I was digesting was from perhaps not the most evidence-based sources.

I was essentially what is now referred to as a 'Bro Nutritionist' – someone who knows a bit about the basics but thinks they know a lot. This situation is illustrated by the Dunning Kruger effect in the diagram below. Sadly, there are many people advising others on diets and nutrition that are firmly sitting at the top of the first peak – knowing not a lot but telling a lot of people about it.

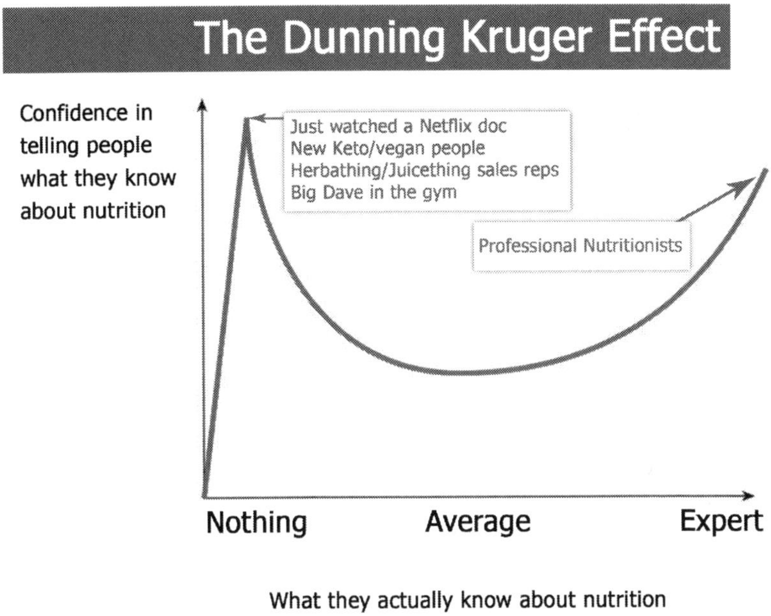

I have no problem admitting my past mistakes as I have learned a million more things since then, and I consistently build on my knowledge.

I knew that certain things worked but not why they worked. This is where most people's nutrition knowledge is based. They know, for example, that if they cut out carbs, they lose weight, but not really why that happens.

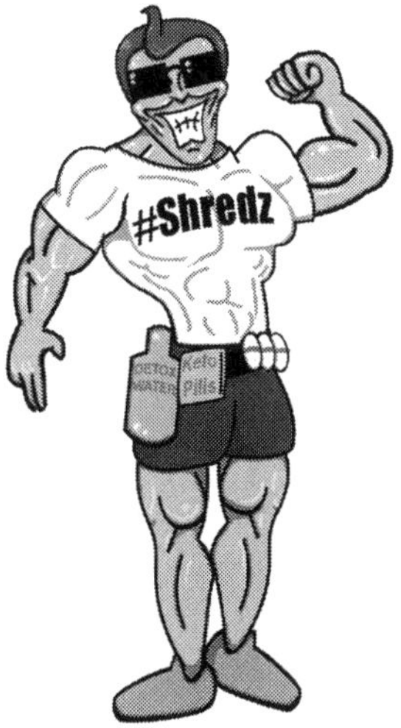

Enter the diet guru, Dr Shredz. He is a fictitious person I created to embody the multitude of bad science – 'abs out, buy my six-week shred plan' people that are all over social media. He's got 100,000 followers, he's got abs, he has the smile and the tan. It would seem he knows about nutrition, as he's obviously living the dream of a tight midsection and sunbeds. Plus, he has 300 likes on his 'diet tea' posts, which he also sells.

Dr Shredz also sells diet plans. He can tell you why cutting out carbs makes you lose weight. In fact, he's got a whole system built around Keto (ketogenic dieting) or some other low-carb thing he promotes and he throws a lot of science-y-sounding terms at you, which seem nice and complex, so you accept they are true and buy his diet.

The truth is that Dr Shredz doesn't really know about nutrition; he has a basic understanding but no in-depth knowledge. He knows what worked for him and that's what he teaches. The problem is that what works for one person may not work for another. Dr Shredz's diet gives the false sense of knowledge that pulls people in, but more often than not it doesn't work for them and they bomb out. His response to this?

"You just don't want it enough."

3. DO YOU WANT IT ENOUGH?

What I've found in over ten years of working with clients for weight loss is that people have varying levels of desire to change; some are steadfast and determined to do whatever it takes to lose the weight, and some need more encouragement but still have that core desire to improve their body shape.

Every single person who has the desire to change can improve their body shape to some degree. They want to take action; they just need to be pointed in the right direction.

What prevents them making this change is friction.

Friction is the thing that erodes our momentum. We start any diet with a full-throttle will to succeed and over time that initial momentum is reduced by various factors that I refer to in this book as 'the friction'.

The friction is the late meetings, the kids being late for school, the shop not having your favourite meal, and being tired on your way home from work on a Friday, which means you prefer a takeaway rather than cooking.

The friction is there every day, we cannot avoid it completely, events will happen. It's how we deal with it that determines if our momentum continues or stalls.

'An object in motion will remain in motion and an object at rest will remain at rest unless acted on by an unbalanced force'

Newton's first law

There are unbalanced forces at work on us every day, affecting our lives. The ones we are competent in dealing with we never really take note of, we just adapt our behaviour to compensate. We balance the unbalanced force; if we didn't then our cars would roll down hills, we would never ascend a staircase and we wouldn't blow on our coffee first thing in the morning.

The forces that remain unbalanced are the ones that mess up our routine. This is generally why diets fail – because there is no addressing of the unbalanced force.

As a former bodybuilder, I have seen countless competitors post on social media about 'pushing through', 'going to a dark place' and 'sacrificing' in order to reach their body fat goals of sub 5%. While I agree this is an extreme diet, and to be successful in any sport you must push your limits, this mentality has translated into the modern-day diet ethos.

This is the Dr Shredz diet mentality; you need to be 'on plan' all the time, which is impossible but still forms the base of many systems. Even if you are allowed a 'cheat day' it's on a set day and for a time-constrained period. Many diet programmes will require that you eliminate certain foods from your diet on the premise that this is the route to success. Others will measure only one metric, such as your body weight, as the indicator of success.

When you start being this specific you are creating extra friction points as well as the daily activities. For example, your meeting overruns, you need to eat something, and you can only get to the local sandwich shop, but they don't do the Keto-approved vegan superfood special leaves that you are allowed. Also, it's Tuesday – you can't eat after 1.00 p.m. on a Tuesday.

Are you sticking to that plan? Maybe for about ten minutes, then you pick up your phone and order an Uber Eats because you are so hungry you've started thinking about killing and eating your co-worker. They are annoying so the meal will be even more satisfying. As a result, you're not even a vegan anymore. You've truly destroyed the plan.

4. FRICTION-FREE EATING

The purpose of this book is to remove or reduce friction. Problems will come up, that's inevitable, it's how we deal with those problems that ultimately determines if our momentum slows or stalls.

In Section 1, I will be detailing the big issues that you'll encounter when trying to transform your body through a fat-loss diet. I'll show you some of the common tricks, and cons, that diet programmes use to lure you in and addict you to their processes. I'll discuss how to recognise a Dr Shredz programme when it's pitched to you. I'll also be showing you how to save money by not spending your pennies on fat-loss supplements that are completely unnecessary.

In Section 2, you will learn about the key concepts in fat-loss nutrition. I'll demonstrate why things happen in your body and why a slowdown in weight loss doesn't mean a slowdown in fat loss.

Then, in Section 3, it will all come together. I will be teaching you how to use all your new knowledge to create a diet that suits your lifestyle. Using my C.A.L.O.R.I.E.

system you will be able to quickly construct an eating plan for a leaner lifestyle that is frictionless and so simple to follow that you'll not even feel as if you are dieting.

I will also be inviting you to keep yourself accountable by letting me know how you are getting on. Posting on Instagram with your completed tasks keeps your momentum going. You may also join my Facebook group dedicated to helping you achieve your personal goals. Search for: https://www.facebook.com/groups/Targetleanlifestyle/

My mission is to teach 100,000 people how to eat awesome food and get the body they want without suffering for it.

Thank you for helping me achieve that goal.

SECTION 1

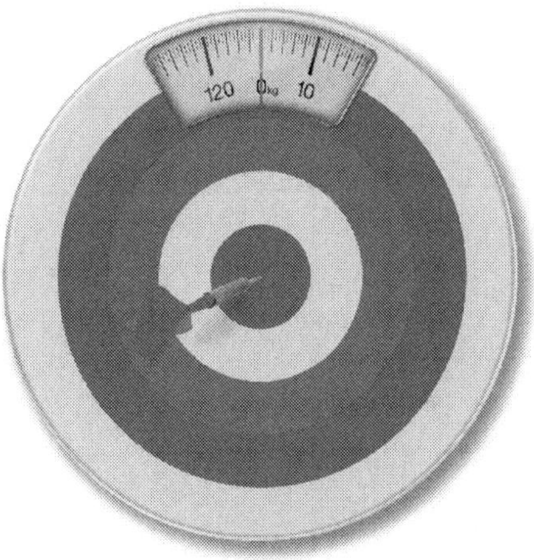

5. THE PSYCHOLOGY OF DIETS

On the face of it, dieting or losing weight is easy. We know it's easy because there's a multitude of moronic social media experts telling us how to do it:

"Just eat less and move more."

While this is essentially the thing you need to do, it is also very simplistic, and you should avoid listening to anyone who is offering this type of guidance as weight loss advice.

For example, imagine if you were an alcoholic and you went to a doctor for advice and they told you:

"Hey, bro, just don't drink alcohol. Problem solved."

What about if you were a gambling addict and the advice from your counsellor was:

"Look, man, just don't bet on stuff. Easy."

Finally, when dealing with serial killers in prison I doubt that the resident prison psychologist's route of treatment is to say:

"You know, it would be awfully nice if you just didn't kill people."

All of these 'solutions' would of course solve the problem if you were an alcoholic, gambler or serial killer.

However, if it were that simple then we'd probably have less of these issues in society.

While it's fairly easy to grasp that addiction to alcohol, gambling, or even murder, is a recognised psychological condition, when the subject of food is discussed this is laughed off by many. Food addiction is often seen as a non-existent or made-up problem. Ironically, we all turn to food as a comfort measure at some point in our lives. However, in other people it is often perceived as greed, laziness or a lack of willpower.

One of the annual social media graphics that I run every Christmas details this premise, asking people not to tell others to relax and overeat during the holidays if they have an eating disorder or are trying to lose weight. It is currently my most liked and shared post ever on the platform.

It's something we see a lot of at Christmas and even more so at Thanksgiving if you are American. It's a holiday of celebrating eating as much as you can, and the amount of so-called nutritionists that are publicly seen to be laughing at people trying to maintain a diet of some sense, is shocking.

While I agree that 'one day won't kill you' would apply to a good majority of people, and I even coach my own clients on diet breaks and calorie banking, for someone with addictive behaviour towards food it's completely the wrong thing to say, despite any best intentions from the person saying it.

Imagine telling an alcoholic that 'one drink won't kill them' at Christmas. You'd soon be going viral on Twitter as insensitive and stupid. For alcoholics, Christmas is a complete nightmare holiday. Alcohol is everywhere and all the adverts and films are filled with people enjoying alcohol, sometimes not responsibly.

I've worked with recovering alcoholics on their nutrition strategies, and the issues they face are immense. Food consumption was an outlet for their addiction recovery, and now that was out of control as well.

I've also worked extensively with people with eating disorders. The triggers and temptations are even more difficult to manage. Food, unlike alcohol, is an essential part of life. We can live our whole lives not drinking alcohol again, but you must eat to live.

Therefore, complete abstinence from food is not an option. Food is everywhere and the shops are filled with lovely treats to tempt us. Supermarkets make the best use of till-side impulse buying and cashiers are encouraged to offer you chocolate deals at petrol stations for a bargain price.

6. IT'S LOGICAL, JIM

To those of us who don't need to lose weight, it can be logical that all overweight people need to do is to 'eat less and move more' to improve their body shape. Until you've lived that life you don't really know the issues that are involved.

Humans are not always logical creatures when it comes to food, shopping, love and Facebook posting. While many of us *know* that we should be ordering the lean chicken with jacket potato from the menu, we generally drift towards the triple cheese pizza.

Why is this?

One of the main issues here is dopamine and it's a massive player in trying to lose weight.

Dopamine is a chemical, which acts as a neurotransmitter in the brain. It's given a fairly bad rap by a lot of people because it's the main chemical release from addictive drugs such as cocaine. You may have also seen numerous articles demonising sugar, because it's 'as addictive as cocaine' due to dopamine release.

However, what's glossed over in the media, probably because it's boring science stuff, is that dopamine is our main driving hormone and it's released in small amounts all through the day. In fact, if we didn't have dopamine we would die. Mice who have had their dopamine knocked completely out barely move all day and don't even want to eat. They have *zero* motivation to do anything. Dopamine is linked to addiction simply because drugs such as cocaine cause a huge release of dopamine after they are used.

What else causes a big release of dopamine? Stroking puppies or kittens for one. Not to say that stroking a puppy is addictive per se, however, I'm definitely a dog person and if any of my members bring their dog to the gym, I'll be all over it and come out covered in hair and slobber. I love dogs and I find it hard not to say hello to any dog that comes over to me.

In fact, I find it incredibly hard not to say hello to any friendly dog, the urge to stroke them is immense. Why is that? I haven't stroked the dog, so I haven't had the hit of dopamine from stroking it.

The answer to this lies in the reason why gamblers like to gamble. They don't win every time, so gambling itself is not the real payoff. Indeed, if the person loses, and it's quite a big loss, then it's safe to say that it's not been a positive experience.

Also, think of this; many people cheat on their partners and then regret it afterwards, however, they may go back for a repeat of the experience many times.

The reason underlying all these actions is that dopamine is not just released after an action, but before. It's not so much the hit of the cocaine, stroking the puppy or the outcome of the bet that drives the dopamine response, but the anticipation of the reward.

The anticipation of a reward from an action will be the reason why a person performs an action. This is crucially important in understanding why people fail at their diets and behave seemingly illogically in their food choices while trying to lose weight.

7. COST AND REWARD

As humans, we are always scanning our environment for food, threat or a mate. Although this is at a subconscious level, it is always there. These are the instinctive factors affecting our survival as a lifeform, and even though we are not really at risk from starvation or being eaten by a wolf in our everyday lives, we still have those instincts embedded in our genes.

In his book *The Hungry Brain* renowned neuroscientist Dr Stephen Guyenet covers many aspects of the hormones affecting the brain, and I'd recommend reading it if this subject is of interest to you. One of the critical theories he covers is something he refers to as the Optimal Foraging Theory (OFT). This refers to our brain's ability to critically analyse the cost and reward of a food. The cost is the time and energy spent obtaining the food and the reward is the calories that you will obtain from eating it. Higher calorie foods carry higher reward values, and the brain will crave them more.

For example, it's unlikely that anyone will really make an effort to search out broccoli and sprouts if they're hungry – they are low calorie foods and don't taste that good, therefore it's a waste of time and energy to make a specific journey to get them.

Conversely, doughnuts and ice cream are very high calorie foods and also taste great, therefore they carry a very high reward value for the cost of the energy spent to obtain them. Indeed, with services such as Uber Eats, we can order junk food with our mobile phones and have them delivered to our house with minimal effort.

It's not uncommon in today's busy working practices for people to go for very long periods at work without eating. The pressure for performance is high especially in many of the jobs in which my clients work, for example, financial markets, head teachers, director and CEO level jobs, as well as shop floor employees on shift work. One of the daily problems they face is that they work very long hours and when they do get time to eat it's a very short window, and therefore because of the OFT described above they instinctively go for the higher calorie options.

It doesn't help when many businesses have vending machines stacked full of high calorie and low nutritional value snacks. One of my clients recently sent me a picture of the table in his office that everyone calls the diabetes table, because of its contents, which are doughnuts, chocolate and other high calorie goodies. Interestingly, they all know it's the wrong type of food for them to be eating, hence diabetes table, but they all dig in nevertheless.

This is an example of the OFT overriding logical thought, driven by the perceived reward value of the foods, and the subsequent dopamine release in anticipation of a nice tasty treat. If people were logical then they'd work out that they probably aren't helping their waistlines by snacking from the diabetes table. However, most people are not logical when it comes to food.

Our reward values are driven by our past experiences. If you've never eaten a certain food then you will have no way of evaluating taste, calories or reward. If you've never eaten ice cream, the image of ice cream on a TV advert will have very little impact on your dopamine levels. There's no real frame of reference for you and so you'll have no desire to eat it and no anticipation of any payoff. Similarly, if you absolutely detest the taste of ice cream then seeing it on TV will also have no effect on your dopamine levels because there would be no reward from eating it.

What is also incredibly important to understand is that the dopamine response to a food cue can override even our own preservation instinct. Epileptics who have seizures, which can be triggered by too much sugar or carbohydrate consumption, still find it difficult to stick to a ketogenic diet because of their love of carbohydrates and the social situations that put them within easy reach of that food. My own partner, Nic, has a gluten triggered condition and she will still eat gluten-containing foods every now and again despite knowing it will cause bloating and stomach cramps.

Cravings and impulses to eat are driven by what we learn when sampling new foods and the feelings and experiences that we then associate with them. Babies pretty much put anything in their mouths as their brains are wired to seek out food even though they don't really know what food is yet.

We soon learn that boot polish is not food, however, that didn't stop me as a child eating an entire tin of it one day. This is a story my mum delights in telling my children again and again. If smartphones were invented back in the early 80s then no doubt it would be popping up in my memories every year, tagged by my mum in a selfie.

Our past experiences construct our anticipations or our best guess when looking at new foods. If a chocolate ice cream is made up to look like steaming dog poo, then we will have real trouble eating it as our eyes will have determined it's not food. The dopamine response to seeing it would be low and so the drive to eat it would be low, maybe even averse to even sampling it. Although logically we know that it is ice cream, it just doesn't *look* right and so is reduced in appeal by our brains, which are getting mixed messages.

Similarly, other senses such as smell and hearing can also trigger dopamine related cravings even when we're not hungry.

The story of Pavlov's dogs is an example of this. Ivan Pavlov was a Russian physiologist who is best known for his work in psychological conditioning. Pavlov noticed that his dogs would salivate when they knew that they were about to be fed. He postulated what would happen if a non-food cue accompanied the presentation of food. He constructed a test whereby he would ring a bell every time he fed his dogs. After a while the dogs would salivate in the anticipation of food from only the bell being rung and no sight of any food.

As humans we are also conditioned to anticipate food from sensory cues. If you ever walk past a bakery and smell fresh bread you will know exactly what I'm talking about. You don't even need to see the bread to anticipate the payoff of taste and pleasure that you will receive from eating it.

Olfactory (smell) cues don't also mean an exact translation of smell to desire for that food. For example, fresh bread means a baker's; bakers sell bread but also doughnuts, therefore the smell of fresh bread can initiate a desire to buy a doughnut. If you generally buy more doughnuts than bread from a baker, the smell of bread may actually give you a cue to eat a doughnut more than bread.

When I was a child I used to love going to the baker's with my mum as I always came away with a doughnut or an iced bun. That's all I buy now if I ever go into a baker's shop, even if I went there for bread.

One of the senses can be a powerful trigger but tie them all together and you've got an almost irresistible urge. If scientists ever get around to inventing a Smellyvision, where the smell of a McDonald's can be beamed into your living room as well as the advert on the screen, then it will be a sure-fire winner for food marketers. Imagine a scenario where the smell of a McDonald's was wafted into your living room through the TV just before the advert was shown, then the next advert after the

McDonald's was one for Uber Eats. You'd have a lot of cues there and also the means of action to easily obtain the food.

The key thing to remember in all of these examples is that you don't even need to be hungry to want to eat food. A phenomenon called hedonic eating can mean that false hunger signals can be sent by your brain at even the sight or smell of a high calorie food.

It's important to understand the difference between genuine hunger and hedonic hunger.

With genuine hunger you'll crave food in a very general way. With hedonic hunger there will be a more acute and sudden trigger of hunger. Hedonic hunger is brought about by a stimulus such as the sight of food or a social event like a party, where you are expected to eat from the buffet.

Therefore, it is important to identify if you are actually hungry or being influenced by other factors before you eat, especially if you are trying to lose weight.

At times we eat only because everyone else is eating and we feel obliged to. One of my client Christiaan's biggest challenges that he faced at his work was that his colleagues would always order a multitude of pizzas for delivery on Fridays. The social pressure was immense and the sense of wanting to fit in overrode his logical brain, which was telling him to stick to his diet plan.

Over the course of six months we worked with reducing the size and design of his pizza from grand pan to thin crust and eventually he decided to abstain and go for a walk instead. What did his colleagues think? They actually applauded him for his over 20 kg of weight loss. In fact, today while I'm re-editing this book before it goes to print, we had a meeting where he told me that a colleague had felt inspired to abstain as well because of his efforts.

It takes a lot of mental strength not to eat when others are eating, especially when this is considered a bonding exercise at a workplace or social event. Not eating creates friction in your mind and the easier option is to go with the herd and pick up the pieces later.

What I want to teach you in this book is to have the mental strength to go against these hedonic cues and make your own knowledge-based decisions. More importantly, you will learn how to override and work with your impulsive brain to keep your cravings in check.

8. THE THREE BRAINS THEORY

You may or may not be aware that your brain is divided into different segments. This book is not meant to be an exploration of brain mechanics, and I am certainly not a brain surgeon or neuroscientist. Suffice to say that certain parts of the brain are devoted to our higher cognitive functions, and some for the more instinctive.

There are many books that deal with the three brains theory. Some refer to the different parts as the lizard, monkey, human, robot, and so on, depending on if it's a business or psychology book. If you are interested in learning more about the brain's workings in terms of our everyday habits and social interactions, then I would thoroughly recommend Professor Steve Peters' book, *The Chimp Paradox*, as it will give much more insight than the nutrition specific topics that I cover in this book.

The three brains theory, as it relates to dieting and nutrition behaviour, concerns three areas, which I will call Muncher, Tivor and Robot. These are all characters from my geek alter ego that loves sci-fi and obscure TV programmes.

MUNCHER

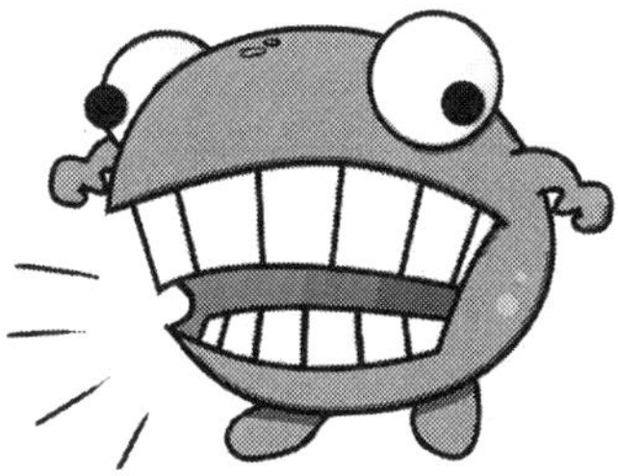

He is instinctive and lives for the moment, his first thought is of food and indulgence and he cares little for consequence. He is emotionally driven and easily angered or upset. However, he cares greatly for Tom and his happiness.

TIVOR
(**T**he **I**nner **V**oice **O**f **R**eason)

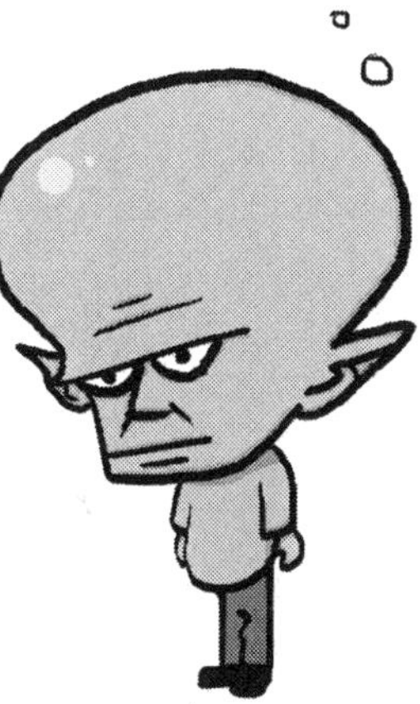

He is analytical and without much emotion. He makes decisions based on facts and logic and rarely gets angry. He cares more for Tom's future well-being than his immediate happiness and recognises that sometimes Tom must endure a little hardship for the greater good.

ROBOT

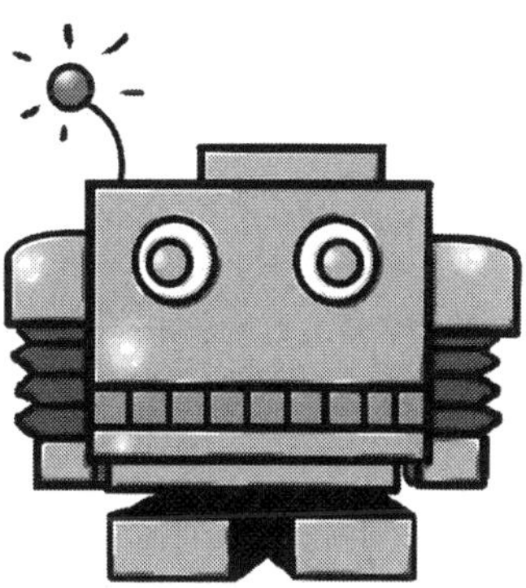

He deals with the day-to-day actions of Tom, such as automated responses to incidents that have already happened and are repeating, e.g. how to open doors and the quickest route to Nando's. Robot is a computer, has no emotion, personality or consciousness and is completely automated in its responses. It does not make new decisions, only what it's been told to do. If it does not understand something it will kick it back to Tivor or Muncher for advice on how to act. It's important to know that Robot doesn't distinguish between what is good or bad, just what it's been programmed to do. Robot is where your habits and routines reside.

Programming happens as a result of forming habits and it helps if you think of this like a computer virus. The virus can be extremely hard to eradicate if it takes hold and can upset the whole functioning of your PC or laptop. Bad or undesirable habits are like viruses and cannot be eliminated altogether and require a 'patch' to restore order.

When you hear people talk about "slipping back into old ways" it's the collapse of a new habit they've formed and the fall-back to the old bad habit, which is still there. You never actually unlearn bad habits, but you can learn ways to get around them.

I've found it useful with clients for them to name their brains so that at any one time they know exactly who is speaking and acting for them. Once they recognise who is controlling them, they can quickly identify undesirable behaviour and stop it. This is a key component to the Target Lean system.

Robot is the quickest and fastest of the brains and if it acts you will be totally unaware that it has done so unless you really think about it. For example, every morning I get up out of bed, brush my teeth and have a shower – Robot will be controlling these actions. I've done them so many times it's now automatic. Any action that is automatic will be done by Robot. This is crucially important as habits are formed by Robot, and both bad and good habits can be formed.

For example, a bad or undesirable habit that Robot may form is always getting a pack of Pringles to eat when watching TV. This is one of my bad habits that I reduced a few years ago.

As successful, lean-lifestyle players we want to programme as many good habits as possible and reduce any bad habits that stop us reaching our goals.

Muncher is less powerful and slower than Robot but faster and stronger than Tivor. Muncher acts on emotion and instinct and rarely thinks about the consequences of his actions, whereas Tivor is slower because he will analyse each situation thoroughly.

Muncher lives off dopamine spikes; it's the brain you use when you dive into the biscuit tin at work as you walk past it, or the brain telling you that you need a doughnut. It's also the brain that gets angry when someone tells you that you shouldn't have another biscuit as you're trying to lose weight.

Tivor is the slowest but also the best representation of you as a person. Tivor is the one that decides to go on a diet to lose weight. Tivor is the one who gets guilty in the aftermath of a bingeing frenzy that Muncher decided to go on before going to sleep in a carb-fuelled coma, leaving you to pick up the pieces.

While I don't expect my clients to become psychologists, it is vitally important for them to realise when Muncher is active and affecting their actions. The vast majority of the time Muncher is taking them on a course that they don't want to travel.

For example, a binge on doughnuts or biscuits. Muncher is fuelled by dopamine, which gives him more power over your actions. It's quite hard for Tivor, the real you, to take back control and stop the bingeing.

Most people when dieting try to use willpower to beat their cravings. This is essentially a stand-up fight between Tivor (willpower) and Muncher (the cravings).

It's important to understand that it's impossible to fight Muncher for long in a straight battle of wills. Muncher will always win as his instinctive drive will overpower Tivor's logical and analytical approach to life. The only time that willpower will beat a craving is when the craving is very low. If you only see a food cue once, then it's quite possible to override it. However, when the cue is presented multiple times in a day in quick succession, the craving will build up and you won't be able to resist. This is what I call a 'Muncher siege'.

If you've ever dieted for a long period, you'll understand that cravings tend to build up over time, eventually resulting in a break of your willpower and a super feeding led by Muncher. And if you've ever been on the receiving end of a Muncher siege, you'll know exactly what I'm talking about.

You see a doughnut; the dopamine release in anticipation of the doughnut reward is high and it wakes up Muncher, who demands that you go and get it and eat it. At this point the craving is low and Tivor can override the urge to eat it. However, if the doughnut is not removed from vision, or suitable distractions are not put in place, Muncher will keep on harassing you. Eventually, Tivor's logic is overpowered, and you eat the doughnut.

Although this may feel as if you are destined to fail on your diet, fear not, as I have a proven system that I've used with clients to keep their cravings at bay by working with Muncher and not against him.

9. BLACK-AND-WHITE THINKING

Life is not always a yes or no answer. Every day we are faced with situations that need a thought about the context in order to make an informed decision about our next course of action.

Nutrition and losing weight are rarely choices between two options. If you are to be successful in applying the Target Lean system, then you need to start thinking in the grey rather than in black and white.

Let's look at an example that I frequently face every day with new clients. At the start of a new diet motivation is high, and you are determined to succeed, so the diet is pretty easy to stick to even if it's a very tough, restrictive one as there's still a novelty factor making it fun. You may make very good initial progress on the diet and lose weight quickly. Then life, in its wisdom, throws you a curveball of a delayed train, or your kids are sick, so you need to come home from work. This creates stress, which begins to wake up Muncher, who starts to suggest that something nice and tasty will make you feel better.

If the stress persists then Muncher's influence grows stronger and you end up eating some biscuits, or potentially bingeing on pizza. The next stage for many is a black-and-white thinking mentality. You think you've ruined your good work from the previous 6–7 days and messed up your diet. This is reinforced by the scales the next day, which show a weight gain.

The result of this is that you may revert to your previous eating patterns, as why bother dieting if you've messed it all up with one weak moment?

Black-and-white thinking is the undoing of many well-intentioned people. To address this potential problem, we need to use a bit of logic.

In the nutrition world it's generally accepted that to gain 1 kg of body fat you need to first have a surplus of 7,700 kcal over your maintenance. I will show you how to work out your calories for maintenance and fat loss later in the book.

Let's put this into perspective – an average man, let's call him Adam, needs around 2,500 kcal from food to maintain his weight each day. If Adam wanted to gain 1kg in a day of body fat, then he needs to eat over 10,000 kcal in that day: 2,500 + 7,700 = 10,200 kcal.

I do know some really big eaters, but even for them 10,000 kcal is a tall order. If Adam binged on a large pizza, then it's likely he topped out at 2,000 kcal. Even if he went all in on some ice cream after the pizza, then he's looking at a top end of 3,000 kcal for the meal. After this he would most likely not eat for a few hours due to the large volume of food that suppressed his appetite.

In one meal it's highly unlikely that you've eaten enough to gain even half a kilogram of body fat. When you get on the scales the next morning it's likely that some of the day's food is still in your system. You may have retained water due to the high sodium or salt content that is generally present in fast foods. Finally, the carbohydrates in the meal have been converted into some muscle glycogen, which can hold three times its weight in water.

The point of this is to illustrate that weight gain on the scales is hardly ever a significant amount of body fat from one day's eating. People get fat from consistently overeating calories every day, which gives the 7,700 figure, repeatedly over a number of days and weeks.

Fat accumulates slowly in the body, which is why we don't notice it coming on until all of a sudden, we can't fit into our jeans. It is a fact that everyone cheats on their diet at some point, despite their initial best intentions.

An occasional deviation is fine, because when we look at the average intake over the week, one meal off the plan is unlikely to have a huge lasting impact. It's important to recognise this and realise that one meal will not make you fat, in the same way that one day's dieting will not make you slim.

Success using the Target Lean system will be from recognising this and not immediately thinking the worst. Mistakes happen, accept them and move on by getting back onto your diet plan as soon as possible.

10. OTHER PSYCHOLOGICAL FACTORS

It's important to work with your brain and not against it. With this in mind there are some crucial things that you need to add to your 'To Stop List' when you try to lose weight.

1. **Telling people you are on a diet**
   Don't ever do this. Most likely you'll get a response such as "oh you're fine the way you are," or some other less-than-helpful comment. Some people will even delight in trying to tempt you with junk food to try to break you. Just say you aren't hungry, or you don't want a food if offered. If people question what you are eating, just say this is what you want today.

2. **Don't ever go *on* a diet**
   This seems counter-intuitive but when you announce, even to yourself, that you are going *on* a diet it immediately implies there's an *off* time. You are setting yourself up for an end point,

whereas a truly effective diet plan will factor in foods that you like in proportion, so that you can enjoy food and still lose fat.

3. **Telling people about your diet**
This is similar to number 1, but different in the very specific way that the type of people that this applies to are the annoying people that go on and on about their super powerful kale smoothie and superfood biscuits that they've made.

Let me tell you a secret: *no one cares.*

Of course, it's totally fine to tell people what you eat, and by the time you've finished reading this book you'll be able to answer any questions about your food with ease. However, I've seen so many people go from being overweight to being slim, and totally bloody annoying with their incessant diet talk.

If you do this, believe me, people will hate you and will hope secretly that you fall flat on your face into a trough of biscuits and regain all the weight. People like humble people. If you find a diet that works for you then there's nothing to say it will work for others, and trying to push your eating habits onto others will not help you in the long run, as you'll close off your mind to alternative methods and become a zealot.

This is how the Keto Cult movement was born. Lots of people telling people that Keto is the best method for burning body fat because, "it worked for them."

In fact, the reason that Keto works for so many people is that the reduction in carbs immediately reduces a certain amount of body water, so there's an instant drop in weight. Combined with this, eating high fat and protein tends to make you feel a lot fuller for longer and so it becomes very difficult to overeat calories. It's still absolutely possible to gain body fat on a ketogenic diet though. Another little fact that you may want to note is that you don't need to be in ketosis to be burning body fat. Many of these diets base a measure of their effectiveness on making the little keto sticks that you wee on change colour.

This somehow is the magic switch that shows you're burning body fat. It isn't. You can be in a calorie deficit for ages before you get to ketosis, and you'll be burning body fat just fine.

Personally, I'm not a fan of the Keto diet for general weight loss. However, it does have some good clinical applications for some medical conditions, such as epilepsy and type 2 diabetes.

I'm an evidence-informed nutritionist. In my opinion, for normal healthy people who are overweight, Keto is another restriction on their lives, which creates friction. The friction contributes to them failing to achieve their goals. I've seen this numerous times in my practice and with clients' histories, and it is my absolute belief that we want to reduce friction as much as possible in our everyday lives so that what we eat is never a stressful or guilt laden experience. Adding in more restrictions, rules and time limits just stacks the deck in your failure and not your favour.

11. THE ULTIMATE PROBLEM

Throughout my time as a bodybuilder and now as a nutritionist, I've come to realise that there are three key influencing factors on a person's ability, or inability, to be able to lose weight and keep it off for the long term.

There are, of course, numerous reasons people cite as to why they can't get the body that they want. In my experience, if you work back to the root cause, it will always be a blend of these three factors.

Confusion, Prison, Frustration.

These three elemental factors often work in sequence, and if you've ever done any sort of diet plan that didn't work, you'll recognise some, if not all, of these factors.

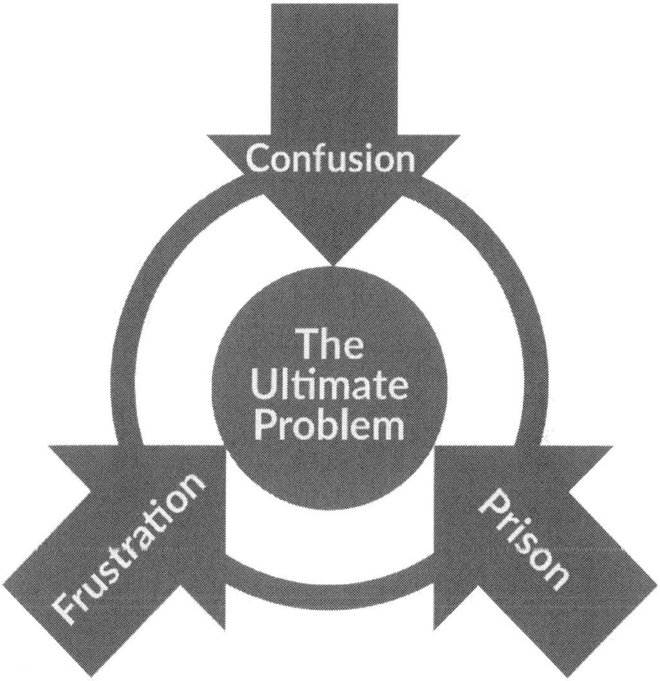
Confusion
The Ultimate Problem
Frustration
Prison

12. CONFUSION

In my time walking this earth I have noticed that you can bank on a few certainties:

- You will always pick the queue at the supermarket that seems to be moving quickly, but as soon as you join, it transforms into the queue where every customer has a non-scannable item and needs Joyce the supervisor to call Terry the manager to "get a code".
- Whenever you drive on the motorway, everyone is a bad driver except you
- Finally, whenever the subject of nutrition comes up, *everyone* is an expert

Nutrition is an incredibly complex subject; I know this as I've been studying it for years and there's still a good amount that I don't know fully, and I'm a complete geek around the subject. If that's the case, what hope does the normal, everyday person have when it's not something they practise on a daily basis?

Of course, anyone can learn the basics. I can just about top up the oil in my truck, and possibly change a tyre if my life depended on it, but everything else under the bonnet is a mystery to me. That's why I always lease my vehicles now, with a full-service package. If things mess up, I just roll into the dealership and they do things to it that make it go again. Magic.

I used to prepare my own spreadsheets for my gym accounts, but it took me ages and then I had to listen to my accountant telling me off for not entering a value at some rate of VAT, or something. I can put things in a line and enter data for accounts, the rest I leave to an accountant, who has actually saved me thousands of pounds and a lot of stress.

I'm not an expert in these matters. It's a professional skill and I don't need to be an expert as I can pay professional people to do these tasks much faster than me and save me time.

Let's apply this to nutrition. When was the last time you heard someone say:

"Hey, I saw this documentary on Netflix on fixing cars, so now I know what the best way to fix cars is."

How about:

"Hey, I saw this movie called Wall Street, *so let me tell you the best way to make money on the Stock Market."*

These things just don't happen. However, we all know people who have watched a Netflix documentary on nutrition and are now experts on the subject covered. Then you have the weekly stories in the press about how drinking a glass of wine is as good as a gym workout, or how rubbing lemons in your eyes helps detox your chakra.

All these stories are taken from research studies, you will know this as the article will always state:

"SCIENTISTS NOW SAY THAT ... [insert moronic statement]."

However, when you actually look at the study that the article is referring to there's a major gap between what the study says and what the article actually says.

13. THE REVOLUTIONARY CARROT DIET

The main problem you have in nutrition is not that the information isn't out there – for the most part we do know how the body responds to food and why fat loss happens. The issue is that you have a huge amount of media misreporting, and social media fat-loss 'experts' that take studies and research and manipulate them for their own gain. For example:

"Keto diets make the body burn more fat as fuel," becomes, *"Keto diets are the best diet for burning body fat."*

I've picked this statement out not because I have a hate of Keto, you'll see me refer to it a fair bit in this book, but because it's something I see and hear a lot of as a miracle diet. While a Keto diet can have some health benefits, it's not significantly better than any others for fat loss.

The real truth is that in a Keto diet you eat more fat as opposed to carbohydrates. As a result, the body switches to burning more fat as a fuel source.

While you might think that this means body fat, it doesn't. It just means that there's more fat available than carbohydrate and therefore the body prefers to use the source of energy that's more abundant in the diet.

You still need to be in an energy deficit to burn body fat, and it's quite possible to gain body fat on a Keto diet. These facts are expertly glossed over with careful language by people trying to sell their own Keto fat-loss diets. You can even buy approved Keto fat-loss sticks that tell you when you are in ketosis, which they imply means that you are burning body fat.

This is just one example. Almost on a daily business my social media inbox receives messages from people who follow my content asking my opinion on the latest 'research backed' fat-loss product. In fact, you can make a diet based on *anything* and providing people are in a calorie deficit, it will work in burning body fat.

You can see an example of a fictional diet video that I have created called 'The Carrot Diet' on my website www.bkmnutrition.com/Carrotdiet, which details how diet gurus use science to trick you into buying their diets.

Ironically, when I tried to run it as an advert on Facebook to show people how easy it is to create a diet to trick people, Facebook flagged it as against their terms and conditions – not because it was misleading, but because it mentioned weight loss. I reworded the ad and it got through. If that had been a genuine ad trying to con people out of their money, then it would have been out there for people to buy.

14. WHY ARE PEOPLE CONFUSED?

Confusion about nutrition is rife across the population and it's beneficial for diet programmes and self-appointed fat-loss experts to keep it that way in order to sell you their diet plans and programmes.

We naturally want to make the right choices about our nutrition. Not many people get up every day with a mission to use the day's eating to make sure they are getting fatter or contributing to their growing risk of cardiovascular disease (CVD).

You don't see many people on daytime TV telling the presenter that they are really happy they've achieved their goal of developing type 2 diabetes. Or how they are thrilled that they need to buy jean sizes that are only made in specialist outlets for obese people.

If losing weight and being healthier is your goal, then when you see a product claiming to be 'scientifically proven' to help you lose weight without dieting, or a food that professes to be low-fat or low-sugar, you naturally gravitate towards that as a choice. What you don't realise is that the low-fat product sometimes makes up its lack of fat with a higher sugar content. Or the low-sugar product has added trans fats to keep a decent shelf life. The calories might be the same, or even more, than the normal fat or sugar product, so it's of no extra benefit if you're trying to lose weight.

You never really get the whole story from the media. The main reason for this is that nutrition is not really a sexy subject, or very exciting. If you ask any of the super-brainy people who teach nutrition education what the best diet is, then they will all say, "it depends." This is where the confusion over nutrition begins.

There is no real absolute best way to do anything in nutrition. The only thing we definitely know for sure is that to lose body fat you need to be in a sustained calorie deficit for a period of time. This forces the body to release its stored energy in the form of body fat for the purpose of prolonging life.

Science has proven this repeatedly with studies comparing all sorts of diets and techniques. Despite this, many diet gurus and weight-loss programmes skip around the subject of a calorie deficit and instead push a specific agenda that they have designed in order to convince you that their way is the *best* way to lose body fat.

Imagine I decided I was going to fix my car's water pump myself. When I looked online for how to do this, I was met with hundreds of sites telling me how to change the water pump, but all telling me different ways. Some say to do it before 6.00 p.m., some telling me I couldn't use two hands, some saying I had to do it using only aluminium spanners. These are obviously very stupid restrictions and conditions, but what if they were backed by science saying that aluminium spanners performed best in a trial, so by this result aluminium spanners should be the only tool used? What was left out was that the other spanners used were rubber and paper.

How about if it was said in the media that Michael Schumacher always did his mechanical adjustments to his own car before 6.00 p.m. – and look at the races he won in his career. The two facts don't relate to each other of course, but we believe from this that we should fix our cars before 6.00 p.m. because that's how he did it. If we fail, then obviously we didn't do it right rather than the initial information being wrong.

This is how we become confused with nutrition and the best way to diet. So many celebrities doing different diets, so much 'science' being thrown at us, and of course there's Karen from accounts who lost weight *only* by drinking her slimming tea.

Important note

Karen also ate less food and was more conscious of her weight while drinking the tea, which is the real reason that she lost weight. An interesting study simply told people that they were in a calorie deficit and they lost some weight. Most likely from being more mindful that they were 'on a diet' and as a result they subconsciously restricted their eating patterns and moved more.

The net result is that you haven't a clue what it really takes to lose weight but are willing to try almost anything that has been 'proven' to work on others.

One of the biggest confusion factors lies in diet plans that classify foods with ‘traffic lights’, ‘sinful’ or even ‘free food’ labels. There are many foods that have exactly the same calories but are classed differently on these diet plans.

15. DON'T YOU KNOW THAT'S BAD FOR YOU?

Classifying foods as 'good' or 'bad' is an inherently flawed process. Food is just food, and it's how you consume it that presents the issue. It's not unhealthy to have a glass of red wine at night, unless of course you are allergic to wine. In that case wine would be quite bad.

However, consuming four to five glasses of wine a night, every night, is probably going to lead to some liver problems somewhere down the line. We all know this; therefore we generally restrict our consumption in some way unless we are addicted to alcohol.

Let's look at one of the most vilified foods – a McDonald's meal. Since the 2004 documentary *Supersize Me* in which Morgan Spurlock sets out to eat his entire diet from McDonald's and developed some very real health issues along the way, it's been seen as a confirmed unhealthy meal.

However, the context of this documentary was confusing. Morgan set out to show that overeating McDonald's would cause health issues, and part of the documentary was that he had to go supersize if asked. Considering that a supersize meal could consist of in excess of 1,000 calories, and he ate 3 of them a day, he averaged 5,000 calories total per day. This put him in a huge surplus every day and he gained 25 lb, or 11 kg, in 30 days.

The health problems that he developed – including higher cholesterol, sexual dysfunction and fatty liver as well as the extra fat – took him around fourteen months to correct.

On the face of it this is a slam dunk for McDonald's being an unhealthy meal. However, let's look at the other side of the story

Ryan Williams, a 29-year-old fitness enthusiast, decided to repeat the McDonald's experiment, but this time staying within calorie limits that are recommended for an average male. He ate just under 2,500 calories from McDonald's every day and lost 16 lb, or 7.2 kg, while decreasing his body fat by 3%. The only major difference between this and the *Supersize Me* experiment was that Ryan exercised for an hour every day, whereas Morgan Spurlock didn't. Now we have a very different picture – someone who led an otherwise healthy lifestyle, lived mainly off McDonald's and dropped body fat. The difference here was the calorie deficit and some exercise.

There have been many research cases involving people losing weight using ice cream, Twinkies and other junk foods.

Anthony Howard-Crow (a YouTube blogger) lost 32 lb, or 14.5 kg, eating 2,000 calories of ice cream, 500 calories of protein supplements, and also a drop of alcohol occasionally. His health markers such as LDL/HDL cholesterol ratio, and blood pressure, also improved.

So, food isn't inherently 'bad' or 'good', but the way that it's consumed, and the lifestyle of the person, can have a dramatic effect on the outcome. There are several studies that look at overfeeding effects in humans away from the sensationalism of the media.

Generally, overeating protein does not have an effect on fat mass, but overfeeding on carbohydrates and fats does promote fat gain. It's easy to see how overfeeding on junk food can be detrimental as it mostly consists of yummy carbs and fats, but not a lot of protein. Remember though that 'healthy' food also contains fats and carbs, and therein lies the confusion. People think that they eat 'healthily' but are actually still overeating calories.

I will talk about how this can be applied to your own diet later on, but as a fail-safe, if you're feeling a bit peckish on your diet then a protein shake might be the best option.

The confusion – take-home message

Don't believe everything you read in the newspapers about nutrition.

Anyone telling you that calories don't matter should be avoided or unfollowed.

If someone is selling the product/supplement they say is amazing and helped them to lose weight, then *don't* buy that product. It's most likely a placebo product and they lost weight from the calorie deficit not the product.

16. THE PRISON

Just before I started writing this book, I was in my local coffee shop with my son, Jacob, having our weekly coffee-and-cake break. Part of our Tuesday ritual back then was to do a long walk combined with a trip to the park and a stop off to have a treat.

Across from us was a table of women, each of them around 50–60 years old, and they started talking about their new diets. As a nutritionist I can't help but earwig on these conversations, as it helps me to understand both my clients, and the sheer nonsense that gets pushed on people by their expert diet programmes.

I don't look down on people who do fad or gimmick-driven diets. I've done my fair share of stupid things to try to lose weight in the past as a bodybuilder. It's a sad state of affairs though, that more often than not I hear people talking about how their diet restricts them instead of liberating them.

This particular diet involved elimination of all gluten products. Gluten is a wheat protein present in pasta, cakes, doughnuts, bread, biscuits, pizza, beer and other foods – basically most of the yummy carb foods. These women were really happy that they'd lost some weight since eliminating gluten from their diets and were discussing how gluten had made them fat. They were also telling the other women on their table that they too should eliminate gluten to lose weight.

I find it hard to keep quiet when I hear people giving advice based on completely wrong information. Gluten is not the issue here; while some people are legitimately allergic or intolerant to gluten, it's not gluten that causes them to gain weight, it's calories.

Here's the issue; gluten-containing foods normally contain carbs as it's a wheat protein and wheat is a source of carbohydrates. Let's look at the foods that these women were told to eliminate from their diet: pasta, pizza, cakes, bread, etc. They are all higher calorie foods and by eliminating them they were removing calories from their diets.

The second point to consider is that gluten-containing foods are also the big hitters in terms of snacking and overeating. Who just has one slice of pizza, or just one biscuit? If you put a pack of Hobnobs in front of me, you'd better stand back as I'll be on it like a piranha fish on a B list actress in a bad horror movie.

Then the third variable to consider is that many gluten-containing foods also contain fat. Pizza is the big one here; a slice of pizza can be 50% fat if you consider the cheese and fatty pepperoni, and so on. By eliminating gluten they'd also eliminated some of the highest calorie and biggest stimulators of overeating that exist in the western diet.

These women had lost weight, and despite being misled by their diet guru, they were happy. The end goal was a positive one, so I was happy that they were happy and it's not for me to interrupt them and potentially confuse them with nutrition facts.

Then this happened:

"I've lost loads of weight, and even better, I've found gluten-free cakes, and biscuit versions of the foods I cut out, so now I can still eat them and keep on my diet."

My heart sank.

These ladies had done so well and now they were about to ruin it all and go back to eating the higher calorie snacks again, which would inevitably mean they would gain weight. The positive change of reducing high calorie foods was about to be undone. In their minds though, they were sticking to the diet as the snacks were gluten-free. The saddest thing about all this is that gluten-free products can be higher in calories than their evil glutenous cousins. These ladies were about to start overeating again, thinking that they were doing the right thing.

Thankfully, Jacob informed me that he'd finished his toasted tea cake and so we left.

17. WHATEVER IT TAKES

The confusion has prepared us for results by any means necessary. Diet gurus and programmes know this. They know that you are desperate to lose weight and they also know that a calorie deficit is what you need to do it. Thing is, if they told you that it was that simple, then you wouldn't buy their programme.

If the solution was perceived as being as simple as:

1. Calculating your calories
2. Allocating them into blocks
3. Listing all the foods that you eat
4. Organising those foods into the meal blocks
5. Routine and habit building
6. Increasing your activity a bit
7. Evaluating the results and adjusting as necessary

Then they'd be out of business fairly quickly as people would be able to do it themselves with a bit of coaching on the seven steps. Instead of teaching you these practical methods, nearly every programme will imprison you in their unique system, which conditions you to their way of doing things. They look to 'addict' you to their method so that you are only able to lose weight their way.

18. BUILDING YOUR PRISON

The gluten-free story from earlier is not uncommon. This type of behaviour is repeated with almost ritualistic precision across most restrictive diets. When I refer to restrictive diets, I mean diets that place unnecessary food or lifestyle constraints on their participants.

Let's be clear on something, every diet needs a calorie deficit to work. You *must* restrict calories into a deficit to lose body fat. It's been proven repeatedly in research and also in some of the case studies that I've already mentioned; calories are the driver behind weight gain or loss.

Whatever diet you choose to do will have somewhere in the small print 'as part of a calorie-controlled diet'. This is the standard small print on any diet food, programme, supplement, detox or whatever Janet from accounts is promoting after she lost 16 lb using it.

Note

You may see that I use certain analogies throughout this book. In my experience, it's generally women who sell weight-loss drinks and powders to each other, and men who push magic muscle-gain pills and shakes to other men. My use of gender examples is simply a reflection of this, and you've probably seen it yourself to some degree.

Like a real-life prison, these programmes all have specific rules you have to follow. These will be based around:

- Food elimination
- Time restriction
- Special days for special foods
- Good and bad foods
- Exercise schedules – sometimes excessive
- Special magic potions, that they endorse and sell. By pure coincidence, see Janet from accounts for details

They will also very specifically focus on weight as the main success factor on the programme. This is what binds you into the prison and ultimately results in your eventual Prison Break.

Life in prison is not enjoyable; due to the restrictions on the programme you are unable to lead the life that you did before. You can't generally enjoy the same foods or social life that you did before, and now you have all these new foods, which are less tasty and not as satisfying to eat.

This is good for a time, as your life before was leading you to being overweight. However, the prison only removes you from your life temporarily and does not rehabilitate you into a new life or identity.

19. ABSTINENCE MAKES THE HEART GROW FONDER

Every diet needs to be restrictive on calories. Later in the book you'll learn my C.A.L.O.R.I.E. method for constructing your own diet plan from calories calculated for your specific needs for fat loss. Before I get to that there are a few things you need to know to make the most of the system.

Calorie restriction is an absolute requirement to lose weight and body fat. However, how you structure your diet is completely your decision. You can be like Ryan and eat McDonald's all day, or like Anthony and eat ice cream all day. As long as you stick within your calories, you'll be on your way to fat loss and a lighter physique.

However awesome a McDonald's or ice cream diet may sound, they are in fact also prisons. We think about diets as eliminating our favourite foods as a kind of punishment for our misdeeds against food and ourselves as the victims. Therefore, we need to be locked away from those naughty indulgencies to lose fat. However, eating only these indulgence foods can also become horrible. Both Andrew and Ryan expressed depression eating these foods every day, and they may have even craved some 'diet food'.

For the most part, people who go on diets remove foods that they class as treats or cheats. Normally, diet programmes will also restrict these items as they are easy wins for the programme. Most treat foods are calorie dense and easily overeaten by people, so cutting them out, like the gluten-containing foods, will reduce calorie intake drastically.

Every time you remove a food from your diet you are restricting your freedom of choice. Normally, it's not difficult to obtain some pizza or ice cream, and it's our decision if we eat them. As soon as we go on a diet and are told "you can't have that," we absolutely want it.

On a logical level, we understand why we shouldn't eat it, but something niggles in the back of our minds. In the first few days it's fine as we are in the hubris of a new diet and our motivation is high. We can do this. We are Sparta!

A few days, or even weeks in, the initial motivation is dwindling, and you may have been at a social event where everyone else is eating your favourite food and you are sitting there with your little salad contemplating your existence. At this point, you may start to realise that this diet is not something that you can do for the long term.

This is the start of the unravelling. Like the women in the coffee shop who had massive success on their initial weight loss, you are starting to miss your little treats and so you look for ways that you can cheat the system.

20. DIET HACKING NEVER WORKS

The women in the coffee shop have found the magic of gluten-free biscuits and cake. They may cost twice as much and taste like cardboard, but they **are** biscuits. Plus, they are gluten-free, so that's fine – they're still on the diet so it's all good.

As humans we are always looking for ways to game the system and turn it to our advantage. In 2018, many Slimming World customers were delighted that Muller Light yoghurts were 'Syn'™ free. In their eyes they believed that they could eat as many as they wanted and did so, sometimes up to 20 a day. The yoghurts contained around 100 calories each and 20 a day would equate to the recommended daily calorie intake for an average woman

Ironically, some were still losing weight, as sometimes they were still in a calorie deficit, but is this behaviour something that you can continue into the long term? Would you want to?

The prison of dieting concerns the restrictions that are placed on dieters without good reason, which forces extreme behaviour and abnormal eating patterns from anyone doing the diet. Eating twenty yoghurts a day may not be unhealthy, but it is weird and it's certainly not a normal eating pattern.

These ladies were devastated when in September 2018 Slimming World reclassified Muller Light yoghurts 'Syn'™ value. They were now NOT free.

21. THE FAKE FOOD BRIGADE

What's more abhorrent is that some of the more popular diets encourage gaming of the system. Ever had a pack of Keto crisps? Vegan bacon? Paleo biscuits? They aren't like the real thing and are arguably taking the person away from the purpose of the diet. I understand of course that people doing the Keto diet may want to have something crispy to munch on, but why not simply show them how to incorporate crisps into their diet in terms of balancing calories?

Paleo biscuits often contain more calories than normal biscuits due to the addition of extra nuts and natural fats, so if the person is looking to lose weight it doesn't help them with that.

Finally, I totally understand why people don't want to eat animals, and ethical vegan nutrition is something I provide for in my practice. However, if you're doing the vegan diet just to lose weight on the misconception that it's somehow better for that purpose, then don't eat vegan bacon. Just eat normal bacon and factor that into your calories for the day.

There are an incredible amount of diets that focus on restriction of calories by proxy in that they reduce calories by banning certain foods or food groups from the menu. This, of course, can cause a drop in calorie intake, until people start to game the system. Exactly like in a prison where people find ways around the confines to make a better life in captivity for themselves, the inmates of the diet look for ways to survive within the confines of the rules of the prison. Until, of course, they decide enough is enough and they can't take the stress or confinement anymore, and they decide to break out.

22. PRISON BREAK

I'm a big fan of James Bond. I grew up in the Roger Moore era of Bond and I absolutely love the classic Bond films. In those films they never really showed what happened when Bond got it wrong and was captured.

If you've ever seen Casino Royale (not the rubbish one from the 70s but the awesome outing by Daniel Craig) you'll remember how Bond unfortunately finds himself in a chair, naked, with a sadistic Le Chiffe baddie swinging a fairly heavy weight with some force into Bond's nether regions.

Suddenly being Bond didn't seem all that great.

Watch any documentary or film that examines torture and you'll be told that everyone breaks eventually. After a while people will say anything you want them to in order to stop the torture.

We can only suffer a certain amount before we decide that we've had enough. Some people have low thresholds for discomfort, and some are incredibly resilient. In the context of diets, the incredibly resilient ones are generally the people I used to hang around with in my competitive bodybuilding days. Competitive bodybuilders have a singular mindset concerning their diets. I've lost count of the number of clients that I've coached for a competition who have told me that they don't care what they have to do, they just want to win. In fact, one year I remember that I would eat cold turkey burgers and broccoli three times every day when prepping for my first Britain outing. The only time I'd eat carbs was at my first meal of oats. It didn't last very long. While doing that I'd also do two hours of cardio a day and train with weights six times a week. Not the most pleasant of experiences and I didn't even win the British title!

Extreme diets are sometimes necessary if there's a short timeframe before the show. I've also had to work with other athletes who have had to make weight for a competition, such as MMA (Mixed Martial Arts) athletes and powerlifters, who've had to really restrict in order to qualify.

The key to this situation is that all of these diets are very short in duration as they are for a specific date. All the athletes undertaking these diets are aware of the finish date, and because of this they are focussed intently on achieving their peak condition for that time. In essence, they know when they are going to be released from their prison. They know when their torture will stop and so can hold out for that time.

In stark contrast, the majority of people in the world who diet have no finish date in mind. They are trying to lose weight to improve their lives and body shape for the long term. The extreme type of diet that creates the prison mentality is not sustainable for the long term, as we can only take a certain amount of sustained hardship before we break.

In an interrogation, this will be spilling the beans about your mission. In diet terms, it will be your mission to spill the beans onto some toast and hoover it up with your face as fast as possible. This is the Prison Break, and it signals your intention to abandon your diet and go back to eating your normal food again. However, normal will most likely be a massive binge to make up for lost time and get all those lovely tastes back that you've missed out on over the weeks you've been dieting. Very quickly you'll gain all that lost weight back again, and you're right back to where you started – annoyed and frustrated that you have, once again, failed at trying to lose weight.

The prison – take-home message

Any diet that requires you to drastically change your habits or eating patterns without a good, explainable scientific reason is a prison diet, and you won't last long.

Therefore, when you eventually leave for either:

- Good behaviour (when you reach your weight-loss goal)
- You serve your time, (the programme ends)
- You break out, (because you simply can't handle any more punishment)

You revert to your old life and behaviour very quickly. A truly effective diet needs lifestyle and habit change to be effective long term.

It's OK to do a prison-type diet if there is a short-term goal in mind, but be sure to understand the consequences of rapid weight loss and gain.

23. THE FRUSTRATION

When I work with clients, I always ask what they have tried in the past to lose weight. There are always a number of usual suspects, which always include the big hitters in the industry. If you've ever tried to lose weight, then they'll most likely be on your list as well. What is the emotion that nearly all of these people feel? Frustration.

It's incredibly soul destroying to try hard at something for weeks and weeks only to end up right back where you started. Yet this is something I encounter repeatedly in my practice.

While confusion creates uncertainty and leads the person to try new things, which end up in a prison of some sort, frustration is possibly the most dangerous of the three factors.

Once you are released or you break out of prison, back in your old life, you quickly revert to your old habits and hang out with your previous partners in crime. Now that you're 'off the diet' you are welcomed back into your old circle with open arms. Despite your resolution to keep up the good work you started in prison, now that you are on the straight and narrow, your environment has not changed. Your identity is still stuck in the old ways and prison was a simple diversion, not a new road. As a result, you have no new habits to follow, no methods of coping with the daily temptations and you are still as confused as ever about the best way to lose the weight that you hate. Without the prison and the routines, there's nothing to help you change.

The result is that you become frustrated and annoyed with your lack of success. You've seen other people get really good results with that programme, so why the hell can't you do it?

If you've ever tried to undo a string of Christmas tree fairy lights after they've been packed in the box for eleven months, then you'll know that the process starts out being slow and methodical, carefully untangling each one at a time, but soon it seems like you're getting nowhere fast and before long you're shaking it about violently screaming, "just *untangle* for God's sake."

Or is that just me?

Of course, shaking it violently doesn't help the situation. Why would it? Logical thought would have told us that, but we don't want to spend hours untangling it a piece at a time, we just want it to be done.

It's the same with losing weight. After plodding along, not getting anywhere, and then crashing out of a diet where the process was horrible anyway, we immediately look for some other diet to follow – some quick fix to get us back on track. This is the violent shake of the lights. We jump right back on another restrictive diet, which is potentially even harder than the one we've just come off. We think that a diet needs to be tough in order to be successful, and that it's our fault we failed because we couldn't stick it long enough. This makes us immediately have another stab at it.

Of course, this also fails to help, and we end up right back at the Prison Break point again. Now we are even more frustrated; we've also picked up a severely damaged sense of self-confidence.

Frustration leads to more extreme behaviour on diets or the willingness to try anything to lose weight. Ironically, when clients come to see me after a couple of cycles on the three factors, and are willing to try anything, i.e. me, they discover that my plan is the least extreme and restrictive diet that they ever follow.

However, before they reach this point, they are extremely easy targets for the quick-fix diet salesmen on the internet, such as Dr Shredz, or the person at their work or gym who sells the latest diet tea or pill.

Frustration is the culmination of the confusion and the prison, magnified many times. Think of it like a spiral staircase whereby the higher the person ascends the more likely they are to have a nasty injury if they fall off. Many people do fall off and end up in massive Muncher binge frenzies – sometimes for months. The belief that they are a total failure and destined to be overweight for their entire life, tragically starts to become a reality.

The person on this journey ends up even more overweight than when they started. Sometimes they take a break from the cycle but then jump back on again before a holiday, or just after Christmas. Generally, dangerous times will be significant dates, such as the first day of the month or a certain number of weeks before an event. Anniversaries such as birthdays or weddings can also be triggers.

Diet companies and gurus know this and will target their advertising accordingly. If you've ever received a letter or email around the time of your birthday or wedding anniversary, it's highly likely it's been targeted for this reason. Normally, it will give you a special offer if you sign up and feature some nice copy about looking better this time next year. All of this is just clever marketing, totally designed to exploit your inherent wish to feel better about yourself and sell you the dream about beating your weight-loss issues.

This book is centred on showing you how to reduce friction in your life and address all the three pressure points. Reducing the pressure points reduces the friction. Once you have no friction you can seamlessly start to change your identity and rehabilitate yourself without the need for any prison, and zero punishment.

Let's start with getting you off the sauce.

24. DIET ADDICTION

The weight loss industry is a funny one as it's one of the only industries where the end goal is to lose its customers.

If you are Apple, then your goal is clear – to sell as many Apple products to your customers as possible, and thanks to the progression in technology you always need to upgrade your product every few years. You generally don't lose a lot of customers if you get the product right for the customer.

Contrast that with the weight loss industry. If you are overweight and want to lose weight, then you go on a diet. If everything goes right, then you lose the weight and you don't need the diet anymore and so you stop being a customer of the diet programme. That's the ideal situation for the customer, of course, but not for the diet programme – they have just lost your business! Of course, they may gain a referral from you to others, but let's stay on track.

Weight loss is big business. In the US, the market was worth $68.2 billion in 2017, a 2.7% increase. According to www.MarketResearch.com growth would continue into 2018 and grow by 3.2% to $70 billion. According to Orbis Research, the global market for weight loss will reach nearly $170 billion by 2023.

It's probably a safe bet that there will always be people who want to lose weight, but if you are a cynic then you might be thinking that it's not in the interest of the big companies, who have millions of dollars invested in the market, to provide a diet that works with 100% effectiveness. By 100% effectiveness, I mean that the customer loses weight and never comes back again.

Of course, they always need success stories. If no one ever lost weight on your diet then eventually people would get wise to it and not buy from you. Or would they?

Depending on where you look there are mixed statistics for people who fail on their diets, sometimes up to a 95% total failure rate. That's an insane figure. Imagine if your iPhone only worked 5% of the time, or your car only started 20 days of the year? You'd be demanding your money back very quickly.

Yet if we fail on our diet, we more often than not blame ourselves.

"I just have no willpower."

"I didn't have the time to prep the meals."

"I couldn't get to the gym."

Diets rely on our brains to be on board with losing weight, and as I discussed in the three brains theory, there are a lot of times when it's not, and it's actively working against our long-term goals.

This generally happens after a period of weight loss has occurred. Remember that as humans we can put up with suffering for a period of time before we break, and so we think that the diet works if we follow it. Therefore, when we fall off the wagon, we generally blame ourselves for our failure and not the diet's structure.

Once we've had a period of becoming fatter again and decide it's time to have another go, we quite often go right back to what worked for us before, albeit for only a short time, and decide to have another go at it.

"Insanity is doing the same thing over and over again and expecting different results."

This quote is often attributed to Albert Einstein, but it's actually from a book called *Sudden Death* by Rita Mae Brown. Whoever said it doesn't matter as much as the message it relays. How many times have you seen people posting on Facebook about going back to [insert popular weight programme], because they have now gained all their weight back? I see the same repeat offenders on my social media feed on a quarterly basis.

25. PLATE-O'S CAVE

Why is it that we repeatedly go back to a diet programme we failed on? Did we not learn our lesson the first time?

Well it could be that, as mentioned earlier, we blame ourselves for the failure. However, there is another factor at play here, our perception of the world and our environment. People perceive that diets need to be tough and they need to hurt a bit to be effective.

The very notion of a diet where you don't really think you are on a diet is almost unbelievable, and perhaps even a bit suspicious. There must be some catch, surely? All the diets you've been on before now involved some sort of curtailment of your freedom. That's the reality you know.

We actively disbelieve people who said they lost weight without much struggle. They are lucky in our eyes, or they have fast metabolisms, or they have good hormones. They are the direct opposite of everything Dr Shredz, in his four-week Shredz plan, says is wrong with you and needs fixing.

A story that illustrates this beautifully is Plato's cave, named after the Greek philosopher.

> In this cave are ten people who have lived their entire lives tied to a big rock in the cave facing a wall, and they have never seen daylight apart from the light that shines in through an opening behind them and illuminates the wall in front of them.
>
> Their perception is that the wall generates the light. They can't see the sun or the outside, just the light on the wall. They all accept it as truth because they can all see it and they all agree.
>
> One day, one of these people manages to break free of the shackles and escapes from the cave into the world outside. In awe of the wondrous beauty, he realises that the light is the product of the sun and he starts to understand the world better.
>
> He returns to his friends in the cave and tells them all about this truth, that the light is from the sun.
>
> He is cast out by the group; they don't believe him because they believe that the light is generated by the wall and they are happy with that truth. They are frightened of this new truth as it's a new concept and they have trouble processing and understanding it.
>
> The escapee leaves the group and continues with a happier life. The group goes back to their life, happy in their understanding of the world.

Think of this in relation to diets. If you've always had moderate initial success with the diet but ultimately failed, then you will be happier returning to that option rather than trying something new. The herd mentality of the weight loss group also convinces you that it's the right course of action, because people shy away from going it alone and leaving their friends.

The perception of diets by the person and the group is that there must be some sort of struggle involved, and you've got to suffer a bit to get results. When they fail, it's because they can't hack it, not because the diet is constructed poorly.

Yet despite their repeated failure they keep on returning. We like what we know, and these programmes become the safe zone for people to go to. It may even be part of the in-group joke that they stand up and tell everyone that they're back because they put the weight on again. Everyone laughs, because they are in the same boat. We like people like ourselves, not people who've lost weight while we can't. We resent their success and then resent ourselves for not being able to achieve it.

26. YOU'RE A BIG FAT CASH COW

Diet programmes know that you'll most likely fail, they have whole sales funnels to entice you back with offers and promotions once you've been away for six months and are about ready to start again.

Of course, you'll lose a bit of weight again, reinforcing that this programme works, however, like before there's no education on nutrition, just guides as to what to eat with a prison of allowed or red-flagged foods for you to follow. You eventually veer off course and leave, only to return in six months because it worked for you last time. You've become addicted to the programme and you don't know how to lose weight without it.

Diet addiction may also involve switching between different diets trying to find the answer to the weight-loss problem. The underlying problem still exists though, you are confused about nutrition. You enter a prison of a diet programme, which you eventually break from and become frustrated with yourself – the three central problems hard at work.

Ironically, the big multimillion companies could very easily solve this by providing an educational element to their programme. With their budgets they could do some nicely presented videos and guides, which would help their customers break the confusion.

So why don't they do this?

Money – plain and simple.

Give people the real solution and they won't need you anymore. Even worse, they might tell their friends how they did it and then they won't join the programme either.

27. THE APPROVED FOODS CONSPIRACY

Am I being too cynical; it can't just be about money, can it?

Please note this is a Conspiracy Theory type story and no insinuation is intended to actual real life events that may or may not have happened and may not still be happening right now.

Let's say you own a diet program and a manufacturer of a food product would like you to endorse their product which was a low calorie food. Using your special made up food classification system you could easily mark this food product with the 'free food' stamp. Your customers perceive it as they can eat as much of it as they want. This leads to thousands of sales of that item rather than another rival brands similar item which contains EXACTLY the same calories. Then you can charge the makers of the food product big bucks to keep that endorsement running. You have essentially just made one food good and another bad despite them being nearly exactly the same in make up and with the same calorie value.

The diet program could also promote their own brands of ready meals and snacks as approved foods when in fact any meal of the same amount of calories would also be fine. This is a business strategy and I'm absolutely not against businesses making profits ethically and legally.

However, at the time of writing I'm not aware of any direct calorie education by the major players that would allow their members to make a conscious choice between a branded meal of 400 calories and another ready meal of 400 calories.

Calories are the reason why weight loss or gain happens. The brand of the food doesn't matter. If the companies educated their clients properly on this then they'd drive away the secondary spend on their approved foods list, reducing their income.

So, tell me again, how do they have your best interests at heart?

If you like a branded, weight-loss programme ready meal, which is 500 calories, but you like a similar Asda meal that's 490 calories but not classed as a diet meal, then you'll be better off with the Asda meal for a weight-loss goal.

28. THE MAGIC SUPPLEMENT FACTOR

One of the most underhand methods that diet programmes use to addict their customers is the magic supplement factor. It's something I have a real personal issue with as it's just a way to rip people off. It's always the same formula, and here's how it works.

If I were to launch a diet programme with a huge budget for the UK, I'd potentially have a captive audience of millions of customers who were totally confused about what to eat to lose weight.

Humans as a whole are impatient and want results quickly. As a diet guru I know this and so I play on it with the magic supplement factor.

I tell people that I have the magic ingredient for weight loss and it's a product called Tom Formula. Tom Formula is to be taken with their specially designed diet plan that I give them, and these two elements combined will give them the weight loss they wanted.

Tom Formula is so secret and powerful that it would most likely be banned as soon as everyone in the diet industry was complaining about it, so really I'm a hero due to me giving this secret formula to you. For a price!

Here's the con though. Tom Formula is basically just some water with some very weak herbs and science-sounding stuff thrown in for extra confusion. The real secret to the weight loss will be the diet I give them, which most likely will be extremely low-calorie so that they see immediate results.

I will go on record right now and state that *every* fat burner on the market that you can buy legally is useless. Most are stimulant based, which is what drives you to be more active and burn more calories, they are *not* fat burners.

Even the powerful drugs that I have taken in the past for bodybuilding competitions did not 'melt' fat off like some of the ridiculous claims of the over-the-counter placebo pills promise. You still have to be in a calorie deficit to lose body fat.

In addition, any product that talks in any way about promoting fat loss, driving fat into cells, stimulating metabolism, melting fat, or any other adjective with regard to making you slimmer, is total rubbish.

There are certain products, which I talk about in later chapters, that might help create the right environment in your body to improve body composition, but none will have a direct effect on fat burning.

The problem is that we do know this on a conscious level; our logical Tivor brain is right there telling us that it must be rubbish. However, we believe the alternative to be a really horrible and tortuous diet without foods that we like and so we take a punt.

This action is reinforced subconsciously by our perception of diets. They must be hard and make you suffer and therefore we automatically assume that the person who's done well has a secret.

It's not uncommon for people who've had success on their diet to be interrogated by the serial dieters as to their secret. Unfortunately, the reply of:

"Consistently eating in a calorie deficit and being mindful of my intake, especially snacking,"

is less sexy than:

"I have been using this slimming tea, which has the leaves of a Slim Tree in it,"

followed by a sales pitch as the person is now a rep for the company in a nice multi-level marketing (MLM) scheme.

Even if the person insists it's down to calories and eating less, we may accept it, but also dismiss it as it's too much like hard work. After all, you have to suffer on diets. It's the law.

29. TYPES OF DIET

This section was going to be a bit of a rundown of all the types of diet and their pros and cons. However, they can all be summarised like this:

The diet:

- Eliminates something
- Creates a calorie deficit by eliminating that thing
- Maybe sells some supplement or special measuring device

Result – person loses weight.

You can gain or lose body fat on any type of diet. The key is always to keep your energy intake from food lower than the energy output from moving about.

There is no secret food that enables you to you burn more body fat. Eating like a caveman doesn't help you get lean. Just because you cut out all meat doesn't result in a one-way ticket to Shredzville, USA.

OK, now that's out of the way.

30. TRUST ME, I'M A NUTRITIONIST

The absolute worst thing about my profession is that it's like the Wild West. Nutritionist is not a protected title like doctor, dietician or lawyer. You can qualify as a nutritionist by buying a £29 course online and completing a very simple multiple-choice exam, or you can invest in a graduate-level degree or diploma like I did costing many thousands of pounds. Both grant you the title of nutritionist.

There are personal trainers telling their clients to cut carbs and drink ketones for performance and fat-loss enhancement – both false.

There are a load of tree-hugging hippies calling themselves holistic nutritionists who've graduated from the school of 'life itself', who will absolutely recommend a monthly colon detox with a kale enema! Thankfully, also false as an effective strategy.

Then you've got people from my former background insisting that their clients eat six small meals a day to boost their metabolism and keep the fires of nutrition burning. Also, incredibly false with no basis in science.

The problem is that all these people are believable. The ripped PT who necks ketones must know what he's talking about. The hippie with the fetish for hoses up the bum must be onto something as she is tiny and looks healthy. Finally, the old school bodybuilding coach has been in the trenches of suffering and torture and lived to put others through it. He must be right.

The first bite is always with the eye. We align to people that are the embodiment of what we aspire to be. Despite my very vocal and blatant statements on my podcast, social media and website, I still get people asking me to coach them on a competition diet. Something that I retired from doing several years ago due to the ethics of some of the methods that I know are necessary to get into that kind of shape.

It's also quite amusing to me that people are quite surprised when they see that my nutrition programming involves dairy, gluten, fruit and all the other bad things that they've been taught to avoid. I guess I should be flattered that I actually still look like some kind of dumb, meathead hardcore bodybuilder, although depending on when you're reading this, I may now look like I don't even lift. A sad day!

Due to the emphasis on how someone looks in terms of nutrition, the battle that I and other qualified nutritionists face is having to constantly unravel the utter tosh that gets spouted by some of these people in the name of selling their cut-and-paste diet plans or their magic supplements.

If a doctor or dietician gave you advice that was not based on science and approved working practices, which then caused you harm, you could sue the pants off them and they'd most likely be struck off the register of the regulatory body.

As of the time of writing there has never been a nutritionist sued successfully by a former client in the UK due to damage from a bad diet plan. Despite there being many instances of people getting truly messed up by these guys, and in some cases ending up in hospital, I've yet to read about any of these cowboys being brought to justice.

Even as a qualified nutritionist I am not able to write prescriptive diets for people, I can only give recommendations on healthy eating practices for a certain goal. This suits my client base completely, as I work on teaching and educating clients to create their own plans, something you'll be doing by the end of this book.

This is not the case for a lot of people. I've seen some very dangerous plans given out by unqualified and unregulated nutritionists, writing prescriptive diets for diabetes and coeliac conditions. This could very well have life threatening consequences.

31. THE CARROT DIET FORMULA

Earlier in the book I referred to the carrot diet, which is a spoof diet video I created to highlight the way that a new diet can be made with literally any food.

The formula looks like this:

- Pick a food or food group
- Make it the focus of the diet
- Reduce down all the other elements in the diet to really low-impact calories
- Add some science-sounding stuff
- Sell to the masses

There are many examples of this such as the potato, boiled egg, cotton wool – yes that exists, cabbage and soup diets to name a few.

Be wary when being told about this type of diet; focussing on one particular food group is not a good idea as this creates another prison for you and is unsustainable. Unless of course you *really* like carrots. Be warned, too many carrots might make you go orange.

32. SCIENCE IS NOW TRENDY

It's now very cool to be quoting science if you work in nutrition, whereas those who have a proper education have been doing it for years as a matter of course. You've now got some serious cherry-picking of research data going on by nutritionists.

Examples of this include:

- Keto dieting for better fat loss
- Supplementing with ketones to improve performance and fat loss
- Green tea for fat loss
- Drinking chlorophyll for alkalising your body
- Various gut health gurus with their magic potions

All of these listed actually do have some studies behind them, but the results are far from conclusive. For example, if you are in ketosis (Keto) then you are eating a whole ton of fat in the day and not much in the way of carbs or protein. This means that the primary energy source that's available to the body is fat. This results in an adaptation whereby fat is converted to acetyl-CoA in the body and then manufactured into beta-hydroxybutyrate, which can be used as ketones to power the brain and vital organs.

However, this doesn't mean that your body is using body fat to do this. It uses the dietary fat that you eat instead, *unless* you are in a calorie deficit, which then means you would need to burn body fat to make up the short fall.

This is skipped over by pretty much every Keto advocate who is not an unbiased evidence-based practitioner. They tell the client it burns fat and the client interprets that as body fat.

Green tea has some research behind it for helping with fat loss. However, to see this effect you need to abstain from caffeine for six months. Six months! I have trouble lasting six hours without coffee. Most likely a high percentage of people who go to the gym, or who have jobs with deadlines, would be in a similar situation. This doesn't stop gurus promoting it and other teas or coffees as a fat-loss aid though.

Ironically, there is an element in coffee called chlorogenic acid that can actually offset the effects of caffeine on fat burning in the body. It interferes with one of the enzymes that starts the process of releasing free fatty acids from body fat. Bummer. However, you still get the stimulatory effects. Yay!

Drinking chlorophyll is a mystery to me. I see so many naïve people drinking it, and there's no real credible research behind it. I'm not sure what they are trying to do, maybe increase their photosynthesis or something.

33. GUT HEALTH GURUS

There's a more recent trend of everyone becoming a gut health guru. The key thing to remember here is that the gut is an incredibly fascinating area of research and it's still very much in its infancy in terms of credible or hard evidence. Even some of the best gut health doctors, with whom I've had the privilege to attend lectures, will tell you that nothing is 100% certain with this area yet.

Despite this, there's a growing number of former PTs who've marketed themselves as gut health experts and used some of the research to state as fact some things that are still not agreed on by actual credible researchers.

One such person has even toured the UK charging £300 a person, per seminar, to extol such benefits as chlorophyll smoothies. Apparently, he alkalises his body in the morning to fight cancer and then makes it more acidic in the evening to kill bad bacteria! The laughable thing here is that your body generally maintains a pH of 7.35–7.45 and actually one whole degree either way means if you haven't died already, you're probably on the way there.

But I digress.

34. STAY AWAY FROM THE WAFFLE

Suffice to say that in recent years, unscrupulous or uneducated PTs and nutritionists have manipulated science to fit their own agenda. This is morally wrong, in my opinion, as it's a nutritionist's job to make the client aware of research and also the potential limitations. It's not to push miracle woo woo powders on them by only giving them a one-sided story to make themselves look like they are some sort of witch doctor.

The take-home from this section should be that nutrition is often overcomplicated for no good reason, normally by people who either have no understanding of the basic concepts, or who are manipulating the science for their own ends. Both these reasons should disqualify the nutritionist from working with people. If you're ever looking to hire a nutritionist make sure that they can:

1. Easily explain concepts to you so that you can understand in thirty seconds why they have suggested a certain protocol

2. Offer both pros and cons of any protocol. This is really important, because even the most basic concepts (apart from a calorie deficit) might not work for some people, and it's important that they recognise this

Always question your nutrition coach. I used to know a guy that would talk at high speed, dropping in science-sounding terms and long words in order to get the client to just agree with his waffle.

I always like to follow Ray Dalio's example from his book *Principles* for people like this:

"If someone speaks too fast then stop them and say, 'I didn't understand that, can you say it more slowly please?'"

Guaranteed if someone's waffling on trying to blinker you, then this will really upset their flow. Ask them to explain each detail, in detail.

I actively encourage this with my clients. I want them to leave me educated not confused, which is what I aim for you after reading this.

If you ever have a question about nutrition, which you think you've been given a waffling answer to, then raise it in my Facebook group – Target Lean Lifestyle. You should find the answer you need quite quickly.

35. CALORIES ARE SO LAST YEAR, HUN

I've talked already about calories and the huge role they play in determining fat loss or fat gain. I do this because I know what I'm talking about. As will any of the superb nutritionists who are my colleagues and mentors in the industry.

A huge red flag should spring up if at any time your nutritionist tells you that, "calories don't matter," and then proceed to follow up that statement with some speedy waffle that makes no sense. This is quickly followed by the inevitable sales pitch into their weight-loss tea or some obscure plant extract, which is the huge secret the fitness industry doesn't want you to know about.

If anyone ever says that calories don't matter on their plan, or that their method somehow magically tricks the body into ignoring calories, then lift your arm, flatten your hand upwards to show them your palm, and if needed, push the flat of your hand into their face to stop them talking. I guarantee that if you don't somehow stop them talking, they will continue. It's easier to be proactive and protect your ears and brain.

36. CALORIES AND STARVATION MODE

Diet gurus love starvation mode. You probably have an idea of what it is, but if you've never had the pleasure of having it explained to you by a complete moron, here's the lowdown on starvation mode, according to diet gurus:

"When the body isn't fed enough, or calories drop too low, the body enters starvation mode. In this mode it shuts down your metabolism and as soon as you eat anything, it immediately turns the food to fat, which then makes you fatter in the long term"

This is normally followed by an explanation that you need to eat lots of small meals throughout the day, to keep your metabolism burning for the whole day, to prevent the dreaded onset of starvation mode.

No one knows how long you can go not eating before starvation mode kicks in. Similarly, they can't really explain how, in places where people are literally starving, they don't enter starvation mode and immediately put on loads of fat once they receive food aid. It seems as if starvation mode only affects people in the western developed world, with regular and easy access to plentiful food sources, who choose to restrict their calories a bit.

Starvation mode has a basis in science in that in a calorie restricted environment the body will downregulate its activity to preserve body tissue. However, in terms of metabolic shutdown this is not strictly true. There is a method of calculating the total energy used by a person in a day called the basal metabolic rate, or BMR.

There are a few different methods to do this but whichever one you use, the BMR will give you an estimate of the calories that you, as an X-amount of skin, bones, muscle, internal organs and water, will need to maintain life. If you were in a coma, this would be your energy consumption.

The BMR is a determinant of life and unless you are going to chop an arm off or remove a kidney, or bits of your brain, etc. then it's unlikely that this will change very much. Having increased muscle does raise your metabolic rate a bit, but it's not mega; an extra 1.0 kg of muscle uses thirteen kcal a day extra to maintain it. Not epic by any means. This also dispels another myth that having loads of muscle means that you can eat huge amounts of food and not get fat, sadly.

What does get affected in a severe calorie deficit akin to starvation is your NEAT activity. This is 'non-exercise activity thermogenesis' or in a basic term, the energy you expend moving around in the day, and anything you do that is not classed as 'exercise', hence the name.

The message of 'eat less and move more' is a direct reference to NEAT and can form up to 50% of the daily energy expenditure, depending on your job and lifestyle. It's also really easy for the body to restrict it by making you more lazy and less motivated to do anything. If you've ever sat and watched a boring programme on trains right after your shooty/action film finished because you literally couldn't be bothered to get up and change the channel, then that's NEAT restriction in action. Or should it be non-action?

Starvation mode is not the thing people make it out to be. Its basis came from observing the fact that when people enter the diet prison, and restrict themselves massively, they slow down after a few days or weeks and as a result the weight loss stalls.

When they break the prison and go on a Muncher binge, they massively overeat. This causes the fat gain. It's not that *everything* they eat has turned to fat, it's that their body has slightly reduced the NEAT, and therefore the total daily energy expenditure (TDEE), and when they binge they hugely increase their calories for a few days, which then causes rapid fat gain.

37. SIZE MATTERS, OR DOES IT? – MEAL SIZES AND METABOLISM

If you've only ever heard one piece of 'helpful' diet advice, it's likely that this will be the one that you've heard:

"Eat little and often to keep your metabolism burning and fired up through the day to help you lose weight."

I used to believe this as well, so I'm not going to belittle or make fun of anyone that does still believe this. After all, on the face of it, it's logical.

The reasoning stems from something called thermic effect of food (TEF). This is the energy you expend to digest your food; a bit like speculating to accumulate, you need to invest energy in breaking down and processing the food you eat in order to get the calories and nutrients out of it. The higher the TEF value of the food the more calories you expend digesting and processing it.

TEF values for foods vary across a spectrum. If a food is more processed, then its TEF is lower, meaning you don't have to take a lot of time breaking it down. For example, mashed potato will have a slightly lower TEF than a raw potato. I wouldn't advise eating raw potatoes though.

The type of food will also determine the TEF value. Protein has the highest TEF and you will invest 30% of the calories you eventually get from a protein source digesting it. This means that for 100 calories of protein (around 25 g of chicken) you'll only be left with 70 calories as a net yield. This doesn't mean that you get 30% less protein, just that you've used 30 calories to get it.

Fat has a much lower TEF of around 5% and can yield as much as 95% of the calories eaten. Carbohydrate's TEF can be between 10–20%, so you can get between 80% and 90% of the calories that you eat from them.

There is a misconception that protein is a fat-burning food due to its high TEF. However, it's important to remember that to burn 30 calories digesting the protein, you've had to eat 100 calories, and so you're still left with 70 calories.

Therefore, trying to eat more in order to burn more calories is a very misguided and wrong idea, yet you still see Dr Shredz telling his clients to do it.

38. SIX SMALL MEALS OR THREE BIG MEALS?

The small-meals protagonists argue that if you are eating a lot of small meals in the day then your metabolism is raised for longer in the day due to TEF, so you are in essence burning calories at a higher rate for longer.

This is only one side of the argument though and there is a key fact that the small-meals crowd either ignore or don't realise. A calorie deficit is determined by the calories that come in from food and drink, minus the calories that come out from activity, existing and TEF.

The thermic effect of food is dependent on the amount of food you ingest. On average this is about 10% of your meal. You can of course calculate TEF on the Protein, Carb and Fat amounts but the time to do this and the negligible difference it would make would be just not worth it.

If you had a meal of 400 calories, then the TEF would be 10% of 400, which is 40. Therefore, the net yield is 400–40 = 360 calories.

If you ate a meal of 800 calories, then your TEF would be 80 calories, meaning the actual net calories would be 800–80 = 720.

If you were to eat 6 smaller meals of 400 calories in a day to get 2,400 calories in total, you would end up with a TEF of 240. If you ate 3 big meals of 800 calories to get 2,400 calories in the day, you would also end up with a TEF of 240. Exactly the same.

Therefore, eating smaller meals has zero advantage in terms of metabolic stoking, or burning, or whatever adjectives Dr Shredz tells you. This is an important learning tool for you to remember when we get to designing your diet plan.

You should feel totally fine with having either three, six or eight, or even just one big meal, a day if that suits your lifestyle better. You can do this in the knowledge that you are not cheating yourself out of any firing up of the metabolism by not going for smaller more frequent meals.

Key Point

As long as you eat within your calorie deficit allowance then you'll lose body fat. This is an important element of choice, which is one of my three factors in a successful, lean-lifestyle strategy.

There was a great study that highlighted this very well and you can see links to it and also a video discussing this topic on my website at www.bkmnutrition.com/big-or-small-meals

Never allow yourself to be forced into a pattern of eating that does not fit your daily routine. This is the prison, which is created by diet plans and gurus and also one of the key pressure points of failure outlined earlier in the book. Such an action will ultimately lead to you breaking your diet plan, and it's totally unnecessary.

39. THE HUNGER GAMES - MEAL SIZES AND FULLNESS

Let's also consider another factor, which is the fullness effect of small or big meals. With small meals you are eating more frequently, however you will have more instances of starting to feel hungry during the day because you must eat within a calorie deficit to lose fat.

Every time you eat a meal you release certain hormones that temporarily abate hunger. The release is triggered by the sensation of food in your stomach and a stretching response it gives. This is short-lived with smaller meals and your hunger soon returns.

Restrictive, low-calorie diets, or ones with miracle fat-loss potions, will also not satisfy you for very long. This can be due to the drastic drop in calorie intake, which causes a rapid increase in hunger hormones. Coupled with an elimination of foods that you like, you can be left feeling unsatisfied in many ways.

When you've just eaten, hunger hormones abate temporarily – you are in the Full O' Food zone. As soon as the food is digested you start to get small hunger signals, which are small at first and then start to increase as time goes on. At this point you drop into the Hunger Games zone where you are not starving, but if food was put in front of you, it might cause you to start eating.

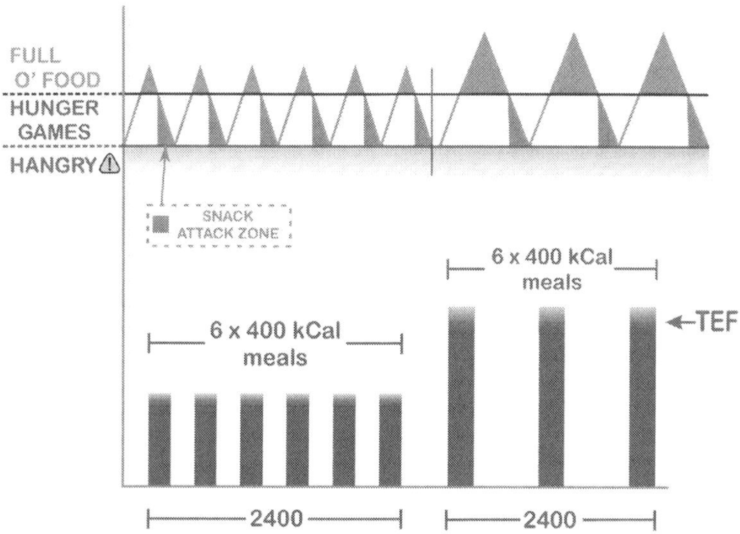

Have you ever been at work and your colleagues bring in a ton of cakes and snacks to keep on a desk at the coffee station? This is where the Hunger Games begin. If you end up eating before a scheduled meal or snack, then you've fallen into the Snack Attack zone, which can be anytime between your meals.

You can see a video and more information on this on my website at www.bkmnutrition.com/hunger-games

This will all depend on willpower and the application of the mental strength techniques that I will teach you later on. People without either of these skills are those that endlessly snack between their 'healthy' meals and then wonder why they have gained weight. Sometimes snacking can also be unconscious, so you may not even remember doing it.

The two main danger zones for overeating on a diet once you are hungry is the Snack Attack zone, where you pick at small items that become large amounts of calories, and the Hangry zone, where your hunger has reached such an epic scale that if you don't eat something then someone will die. Then you might eat them.

It's easier than you think to slip into the Hangry zone. Say you have six small meals planned out in the day and at meal two your meeting overruns so you miss the meal and go another hour without eating. Then when you get out there's a phone call or deadline you need to hit before the lunch hour. Quite quickly you're missing out on two meals and because you only ate a small meal earlier, you're very quickly descending into Hangryness.

You get a ten-minute break and now that your hunger has reached such epic levels, your optimum foraging instinct – from the Optimal Foraging Theory (OFT) – kicks in. Instead of the balanced and healthy two meals you were going to have, you dash out and find the highest calorie quick-snack you can, which is the local Greggs or garage for a meal deal that you can demolish in thirty seconds. While this does satisfy your hunger, the food is overly processed, which means it's digested quickly and doesn't keep you full for long, so you're back to the escalating Hunger Game for the afternoon.

Although this admittedly is a very specific situation, it's merely to highlight that life does not go to plan and our best laid plans can quite quickly go to ruin from events outside of our control.

Unless you have the cognition to bunch your small meals together into one big meal, which would be a Tivor action, then you will most likely fall foul of the vengeance of your Hangry self, which awakens the Muncher brain in you. Muncher fights for your survival on instinct. The instinct tells you to seek out high calorie food very quickly, and so you override your logical brain, which results in a mini binge of calories.

For some people this then opens the floodgates for the day seeing as they've gone off their diet, they proceed to go off it for the whole day, vowing to, "get back on it tomorrow."

40. IS IT MORE BENEFICIAL TO HAVE BIGGER MEALS?

The argument for bigger meals is based around being in the Full O' Food zone for longer after a meal. If you've ever had a really big Sunday dinner with your family, then you'll know the feeling of being so full that you may not eat for a good few hours or even again for the day. The incredible amount of food that has maxed out your full hormones, coupled with your initial view of the meal as a big volume of food, keeps your hunger at bay for a good amount of time.

Staying full as a sensation has its advantages of course, in that your mind isn't on your food, so you are free to focus on your work or whatever you're doing in the day. If you have to break for meals every two hours, then it can disrupt your workflow.

When writing this book, I generally ate a very large breakfast and then ate nothing for the whole morning while I wrote the book in various coffee shops dotted about Bristol, and sat at the bar on my holiday in Greece.

The idea was to keep my mind firmly on the task at hand. If you've ever had a big project to get finished, you'll understand how hunger can distract your mind and actually prevent you doing your best work.

Many of my clients also find the big-meals approach beneficial, as they have days that are stupidly busy with meetings that drag on, or huge projects that can take up a whole day to get finished for a deadline. Before they worked with me, they'd gone down the little-and-often route and face-planted dismally into takeaways and Uber Eats delivered to the office.

Finally, the prep time for lots of little meals can be time-consuming. Give someone a big breakfast, one very big lunchtime meal and a big evening meal and they have very little to think about. A lot of my clients avoid breakfast completely, or have a very small snack, then fast until after 1.00 p.m. They have a bigger lunch, then a big evening meal with their family. This fits their lifestyle perfectly and they are very successful with their weight-loss goals as a result.

Let's be clear here though, the big-meals scenario does allow for small nibbles through the day, and I always set aside some snack calories. To give a brief explanation, if you don't have a snack allocation in your calories then you'll still end up snacking, but it will be in the Snack Attack zone, which is unregulated and takes you outside your calories for the day. By defining and allocating snacks you allow yourself a choice to have, or not have, the extra calories and be in a deficit in both instances.

When I say snacks, I don't mean carrot sticks or celery, I mean proper allocations like Halo Top ice cream and things you actually like to snack on. In an ideal situation I'd like to say to my clients to have very low-calorie and healthy snacks, however, it's unrealistic that they'll like eating this on a regular basis. Many of my clients allocate a certain number of calories to their snacks, and create a list of snacks to fit those calories. This way they have options if they have to go to a local shop between meetings.

In theory, the big-meal option allows you to go longer before getting hungry and gives you more latitude with your meals. If you know you've got a sizeable meal coming up, you can hold out a bit longer in order to enjoy a good feast. Holding out for a smaller meal isn't such a tempting prospect.

I am an advocate of bigger, less frequent meals, but this is more to do with my personal circumstances. Remember that you should always eat around your lifestyle.

Whichever avenue you choose, make sure it's one that is best for you, not one that's given to you by your guru diet person with abs. If they can't build you a diet based around your lifestyle then they aren't much good to you and are probably giving you the same plan they gave the other ten people that signed up to their 'Strong and Lean' style twelve-week plan.

Of course, if your lifestyle is three takeaways a day and four pints of lager every evening, then you probably *should* adjust that lifestyle. With all my skills as a nutritionist, I just can't make that stick as a weight-loss plan in any way.

I did have a client like that once, and we worked really hard to get his bad eating habits down to only one low-calorie beer a night while switching to low-fat and lower-calorie ready meals from the supermarket. These were small adjustments, but the drop in calories was enough to see a 15 kg weight loss result, which he was happy with. He never got to a visible six-pack, but that's not what he wanted. Just not being prediabetic, able to get into much smaller clothes and begin a relationship with the girl he fancied was his target.

Remember that targets should be achievable. Six-packs take a lot of effort and dedication and in most cases require a very restrictive calorie intake with lots of exercise. But you *can* do it with big meals or small ones.

41. SHOULD YOU REDUCE YOUR CARB FOOTPRINT?

Overwhelmingly, one of the biggest issues I deal with as a nutritionist and fat-loss coach is the commonly held belief that carbohydrates are the cause of people's fat gain. When people decide to go on a crash diet the first thing most do is cut out carbs. This does tend to work in the short term because they have cut down on calorie intake. As you are hopefully starting to understand, it's calories that are the main driver in weight loss, or more specifically, a calorie deficit.

Reducing carb intake would be an effective method *if only people could stick to it*. Most people really like carbs and after a while they start to miss all the great carby goodness from their previous diet. You have probably been there yourself and cut carbs out for as long as you could before failing miserably and face-planting into a huge bowl of cereal, which turns into an epic rampage of sugary decadence.

Key Point

Remember that eliminating a food group or drastically reducing it is part of a prison and the prison always results in a Prison Break. Unless you start to really enjoy eating only protein, veg and fats, it's likely that a zero, or very low-carb lifestyle, will be a miserable one.

You may have tried the zero or low-carb approach before. I have – many times for bodybuilding competitions. I rampaged through carbs once the show had finished. After the British finals one year I sat in Pizza Hut eating flapjacks waiting for my pizza to arrive. Insane behaviour.

Although low-carb diets can be effective, I want to give you some ideas as to why they are not necessarily the right choice.

I want to add some 'it depends' caveats here. People who can really benefit from low-carb diets include:

- People who exercise very little and are generally couch potatoes with little movement. If that's you, then I do suggest that you look to change this, or you may end up in the next criteria
- People who have pre- or type 2 diabetes who want to reverse the condition. Lower carb intake can increase their insulin sensitivity and help to prevent the build-up of glucose in the blood or the accumulation of body fat from *de novo lipogenesis*, which is when carbs turn to fat
- People with epilepsy. Keto or very low-carb diets can go some way to reducing seizures in some cases

- Women with polycystic ovary syndrome (PCOS)
- People who enjoy Keto – weird but I don't judge

I would stress here that you should always consult your doctor or dietician before changing your diet, which may be specific to your condition.

For anyone else there's no real reason to eliminate carbs from your diet and you should be able to enjoy them in moderation, which means within your maintenance or calorie deficit.

Notice I don't include people who are gluten intolerant here as gluten is a wheat protein that exists in wheat source carbohydrates, such as wheat, obviously, bread, most pastries and cakes.

Rice, oats (generally) and potatoes are usually OK to eat. In the same way as reducing carbs reduces calorie intake, going gluten-free only serves to reduce calorie intake, which then helps with fat loss. Unless of course you substitute normal muffins for gluten-free muffins, then you've just calorie swapped.

Let's also look at some key points for carbohydrates.

1. Carbs are the key source of energy for the muscles, and if you train with weights you will be using stored carbs in the form of glycogen to exercise with. When you do this your body tries to replenish your glycogen stores as fast as possible, so if you train and then eat a big carb meal it's unlikely that you'll store any carbs as fat from that meal.

2. Carbs contain 4 calories per gram whereas fats contain 9 calories per gram, which means you get twice as many calories for your money over fats. This also means that your food volume from carbs can be higher resulting in a fuller feeling. This is very important as many people will swap their carb snacks for nuts, which are 50% fat and much higher in calories per 100 g. A good handful of nuts can be as much as 250 calories. Therefore, dropping carbs and swapping to 'healthy' snacks may actually result in you overeating. Of course, I'm not saying don't eat nuts, as they contain great micronutrients and unrefined fats and fibre, but it's important to take the calories into account if you're trying to lose weight.

3. Carbs don't really turn into fat that well. One overfeeding study found that on average only 10% of the calories from 1,000 calories of carbs (250 g) that were overeaten ended up as body fat. That's around 9 g of body fat from 250 g of carbs, which is just over 1 kg of potatoes or 300 g of rice. Fat on the other hand converts to body fat very easily. That's not to say you won't get fat eating carbs, but it's less likely than if you're overeating fats as a main food source.

4. There's a myth that fruit turns to fat easily. Wherever this came from originally, a recent study found that only around 1% of fruit sugar ends up as fat. Fruit should be far from the first thing you drop from your diet. Both the fibre

and nutrient profile of fruit make it a great addition to your diet as well as the low-calorie yield per 100 g. Blueberries, for example, are around 40 kcal per 100 g. That's low.

5. In studies where the calories were matched, and the variables were carb and fat amounts, there was little to no difference between a higher-fat or higher-carb diet. Evidence that carbs themselves are probably not the reason for fat gain.

You might get the feeling that I'm a pro-carb person. I'm actually not, and despite my best efforts, I'm pretty rubbish at eating a lot of carbs, which is sort of a bad thing when you're a bodybuilder. I'm not pro carbs, I'm just anti stupid. I see so many gurus and idiotic articles in newspapers saying completely wrong things about carbs that I feel the balance should be addressed. The fallout from this type of silly scaremongering is something I deal with every single day.

Case Study – Hazel's fear of carbs

Hazel was a client who came to me with a severe fear of carbs from years of being in the prison state of mind, fuelled by frustration from failing to lose weight despite being on very restricted diets. She had developed a mixture of eating disorders, which were ruining her life and taking over her behaviour.

We determined that the root of all this was the confusion around nutrition that led her to the belief that carbs were the evil that was driving her weight gain. With all three pressure points exerting a heavy influence she was feeling the stress.

Hazel was not a stupid person, in fact, far from it. She had a high-powered job as a project manager for a big company. She was highly intelligent and motivated but had become blinded by the mixed messages. She also would occasionally go off her diet and this would result in a binge, which she then would beat herself up over with extreme cardio activity and further food restriction.

The first step was to explain clearly that the root cause of weight gain would be her calorie intake and more importantly her average intake over the week, so that one bad day didn't matter in the grand scheme. Once we had laid out all the basics, we set to constructing a plan that slowly introduced moderate amounts of carbs, while still keeping a calorie deficit on average over the week.

Hazel started seeing results quite quickly after this and and we reduced her cardio from hours a day to hours a week while giving her weight training a kick-start. This required more carbs and with the results really starting to show, she was willing to go against her ingrained belief that carbs would make her fat.

Over the course of a year Hazel dropped her body fat to nearly single digit percentages and increased her muscle mass. Moreover, she's now enjoying carbs with most meals and her fear of being photographed has gone. In addition, her reliance on the scales as an indicator of progress is now non-existent. She knows that muscle gain will result in more glycogen and water held in the muscle, which may make her a bit heavier.

All Hazel's problems stemmed from the confusion about nutrition. This had cascaded into the prison and frustration. At the root of this was a belief that carbs were the enemy. In fact, they have become her friend now and while she still has to control intake and limit certain foods that trigger bingeing, she's a lot happier with herself and much more confident.

42. BIG FAT LIES

Fat has had a rollercoaster ride in recent years. It used to be the evil nutrient that you had to stay away from as much as possible. More recently though it's become more trendy to have a higher fat content in the diet and the Keto diet, or very low carb diet (VLCD) is making a real comeback.

As I write this book there are more Keto gurus online than I've ever seen before. A great many of them continue to promote a very wrong idea that eating more fat promotes body fat being used as fuel. It's an easy hook for people to swallow and it's kind of based in science. If this was a scientific paper, I'd quote all the studies, referencing ketones in sports and their application, as well as the keto adoption athletes. However, I'm taking a guess that the majority of my readers are either other nutritionists or professionals who know the studies I refer to, or people like my clients who don't care about the nitty gritty and are happy with a brief synopsis so they can tell Derek in their office to stop trying to sell them keto salts.

Here is a brief overview.

Your body prefers to burn carbohydrates for exercise for the most part unless it's very slow in output, e.g. walking. Even professional marathon runners burn mostly carbohydrates for fuel because the intensity they run at is so fast that fat cannot be turned into ATP (adenosine triphosphate, the body's energy source) fast enough.

However, there are certain times that the body can switch to using fat for fuel as a primary source and one of these situations would be when you have a very low carbohydrate diet.

Without carbs as an abundant fuel source the body can become what's referred to as 'fat adapted' and turns fat into ketones as a survival measure so that the brain and internal organs, which rely on carbs primarily as fuel, can continue to function optimally.

In essence, the body is burning more fat for fuel. The *big* thing that must be remembered here is that in a ketosis diet, where carbs are very low, the fat content of the diet is incredibly high, almost 70% of the calories will come from fat. If we were to look at the recommended calorie intake for a female at 2,000 calories a day, that's 1,400 calories from fat or 156 grams. To put that into perspective that's about half a can of coke's worth of olive oil.

With so much fat in the diet, and so few carbs, the body logically switches over to using fat as a primary fuel source in order to conserve what little carbs are available for high-intensity exercise. This is what keto conmen have latched on to and sell a Keto diet as one that burns more body fat as fuel. In fact, the majority of the fat that is burned will be from the dietary fat that the person eats.

Key Point

It's crucial to remember that whether in a low-carb or low-fat scenario, the determining effect on body fat burning will be the calorie deficit that the person creates. As a rule of thumb around 7,700 kcal of deficit will elicit 1 kg of body fat burned. This has been studied extensively and only a fool or someone trying to con you will tell you that calories are unimportant compared to the fat or carb make-up of the diet.

Another nice con trick in recent years is the selling of keto salts as a fat-loss agent. These products contain the simple salts that the body manufactures from fats in ketosis. Keto gurus will tell you that this will put you into ketosis and they show you that you are doing this by measuring ketones in your urine. Ketones that you've just eaten.

Ironically, the research on ketone salts in its early stages shows that it actually impairs performance from inhibiting carbohydrate use as fuel. My advice is to stay clear of this overpriced and potentially worthless supplement.

43. THE PROTEIN AVENGER

If any macro was to save the world it seems that protein would be it. It used to be just bodybuilders that held the flag high for increased protein intake and for years the non-bodybuilding muggles laughed at them for chomping down buckets of this muscle-building nutrient. However, in the last five years or so as if from nowhere, suddenly everything is *protein*.

Whether it's because we are becoming more health conscious as a population or the seemingly now acceptable practice of having a visibly muscled body – thanks, in part, to The Marvel Universe – products that would never before be associated with muscle building now have added protein.

It used to be that protein bars and snacks were the preserve of the supplement companies that churned out chalky tasting bars with some whey added to them. Today that's not the case. What started with Quest, and now the market dominant Grenade bars in the UK, has cascaded into a protein army of foods and drinks that vie for our money.

Protein coffee, Weetabix, cornflakes, Snickers bars, even crisps now have added protein to try to tempt the consumer into purchasing them for their muscle-building efforts.

As with all these gimmick products there is a catch. The protein they add is generally pretty crap at building muscle.

Protein is composed of twenty-two amino acids, and seven of these are what's classed as essential in that the body cannot make them itself and so must get them from the food that you eat. The main essential amino acid responsible for muscle building is called leucine.

To make the process easier to understand I want you to think of leucine as the light dimmer switch in a room. Once you turn it on you can turn it up to a certain level, but after a few turns the light doesn't get brighter even if you turn it more. Leucine has a dose-dependent effect on the body and more doesn't equal better results once a threshold has been reached.

The other six essential amino acids support the effect of leucine and so you can think of these as the electricity behind the light switch. Without the initial turning on by the leucine the other essential amino acids won't have an impact on muscle-building signals. Similarly, without the support of the other amino acids, the initial signal from leucine will quickly disperse, same as the way a light in a room may turn on for a second but without power will fade out very quickly.

Why is all this relevant? Most of the protein added to these 'protein' products is completely worthless for enhancing muscle building or any fitness related benefit. In fact, more often than not it's a pretty worthless gluten-based protein. That's right, gluten. The evil carb protein that a lot of people are afraid of.

Even more of a disappointment is that most of these protein products have very minimal amounts of added protein in, one of the chocolate bars advertised as 'protein' actually only had 2 g more protein than its normal counterpart, but the price tag was a pound more expensive. You could actually get a better protein dose from a small glass of milk, which costs about 50p and actually has leucine and all the amino acids in.

Here's my advice on the protein products. If something is not inherently a protein food, such as chicken, eggs, beef, lamb, turkey, milk, whey, fish, or one of the vegan/vegetarian sources with added aminos such as seitan, tofu, Quorn, edamame, etc. then it will not benefit you as a protein food. Even protein bars need to be treated with caution. Check the source on the back as if it contains a lot of collagen, which some do to bump up the protein content cheaply, it is less effective at building muscle.

Imagine I tried to sell you some 'Carb Chicken', which was chicken with some added potato starch in. How about some 'Fat Cornflakes', which was cornflakes with added olive oil. Both of these products cost twice as much as the normal version. You'd tell me to jog on. If you wouldn't, then please email me immediately with the subject title 'sell me tat' as I've got a load of stuff I can palm off onto you from my Del Boy suitcase.

If you want to add more protein to your diet, and actually reap the benefits of a higher-protein diet, then eat or drink more actual protein-based foods. In the same way that chicken flavoured crisps aren't a beneficial protein meal, protein chocolate bars or breakfast cereal will not change your life for the better.

44. 'WEIGHT' A MINUTE – WHY THE SCALES SHOULD NOT BE THE ONLY JUDGE

The scales can be both an ally and your enemy. One day they are showing you how much weight you've lost, the next they are saying you've put on a few kilos. For those trying to gain muscle they'll accept any movement up as a bonus, even if it's fat. For those trying to lose body fat, they'll accept any number that's less than the previous day's value.

The issue with always watching the scales as an indicator of progress is that muscle gain does not happen very quickly, and fat does not drop off very quickly. Muscle takes months and months to accumulate to any great degree if you are natural (not taking anabolic steroids) and even if you are using drugs to accelerate the gains then it's still not going to be ground-breaking. Fat can drop off at a quicker rate than muscle accumulates, but it's still not a huge shift.

Key Point

As a rule of thumb, you need to be in a deficit of 7,700 calories to drop 1 kg of body fat, and even if you hit that number it's not guaranteed to be all body fat. The body is made up of over 70% water and changes in hydration status can deliver a quite sizeable swing in your body weight.

You also have to remember that 7,700 calories is a massive number and it's unlikely you'll hit this deficit in a day unless you've run a few marathons and not eaten at all that day, in which case you're likely dead or close to it so fat loss isn't your first concern.

Conversely, it's entirely possible to hit 7,700 calories over your maintenance to potentially gain a kilo of fat in a day, but that would be some serious eating. One of my best friends, Dr Emil, used to drink olive oil to gain weight as fast as possible for strongman events, but I definitely wouldn't recommend this as a daily nutrition plan. For most people eating 7,700 over their maintenance amount would push their daily calorie intake up to 9,500–10,000. That's a seriously determined effort.

If it's not fat or muscle, then what is the cause of a major shift in weight on a day-to-day basis?

Exhibit A: Glycogen and rapid weight gain

Glycogen stored in the muscles can cause a swing both ways. Glycogen is the stored form of carbohydrate in the muscle and liver and in a normal person this can be about 500 g. Glycogen can hold up to three times its weight in water. If you are fully loaded with glycogen you may be 2 kg heavier – 500 g x 4 = 2,000 g/2 kg.

As you exercise you will use a mixture of glycogen and fat to fuel your activity; this depends on the intensity of the exercise. More intense exercise leads to more glycogen over fat being used. You'll also release water from the glycogen that you use. This will cause a drop in weight from water excretion and a drop in glycogen stores, but there's no impact on body fat or muscle levels.

When you eat after exercise, your glycogen stores will be replenished over time but depending on when you choose to weigh yourself this may be before, during or after the process, so you'll get different body weights.

Exhibit B: Hormone changes

Other conditions in the body may also cause a retention of body water such as high sodium, or a reduction in diuretic hormones, or if you have underlying kidney issues that prevent the excretion of water. If you're a woman then you'll know that water retention associated with a rise in progesterone and oestradiol can occur around or just before your period.

Exhibit C: Food

The third condition just may be the amount of food in your system. Depending on how efficient your digestion is you can have up to forty-eight hours of food in your system. This contributes to your overall body weight. Fibre such as vegetables will also slow down digestion to a degree, which can lead to retention of weight. I've also had clients reporting eating a ton of roasted dry veg only to have it bloat them hugely.

This is a very important consideration when I help athletes with making weight for competitions in boxing or powerlifting. They still need to eat, but the margin can often be so tight that we need to make sure the foods eaten are light in weight as well as providing the necessary calories.

For example, ice cream from McDonald's can be a very light but dense source of calories, so ideal as a pre-fight boost when weights are literally down to the gram. Rice cakes are also a good source of volume in terms of filling the person up and abating hunger without providing much weight as they are generally 50% air.

Chicken breast and brown rice would be a very heavy meal in comparison and may put the athlete over their limit. Therefore, when stepping on the scales, it's really important to consider what you've eaten in the last twenty-four hours and how active you've been.

Generally, people will be heavier on a Monday because they eat a bit more at the weekend and do less. Conversely, they will be lighter as a rule on Friday morning after a week of exercise and work routines. It's important that you know this as your first action on a Monday might be to step on the scales and that may start your week off with a negative undertone that could seep into your work and family life.

However, despite knowing all this, and however fervently Tivor tries to convince us that it's just a blip, Muncher immediately rises up to our aid and generates cravings for some nice food to calm our nerves. After all, we have already gained weight so what's one cream cake going to matter?

This is an effect from the confusion of not knowing why the weight is fluctuating, leading potentially to a break from your diet plan via frustration at your apparent lack of progress. However, in most cases it's only a temporary factor. If we recognise that weight is a fluctuating factor and instead look at the weekly average, then we get a bigger picture.

Logging your weight every day might be considered a little over-controlling. Others argue that it brings the focus onto the weight as a success measure. This might be the case if the person was not educated in the reasons behind weight fluctuation, but you now should be aware of all those potential issues.

Weight should only be one factor in your determinants of progress. I normally ask clients to log their calorie intake, their steps and their exercise as well as their weight so that we have a broad measure of total calories in and calories out (CICO). When you have a big picture, you can then make an informed decision about where the potential issues might be and adjust your lifestyle accordingly. Did you notice I didn't say "adjust your diet"? That's because the vast majority of the time adjusting your diet is not the right course of action.

More often than not when I sit down for a weekly check in with my clients, we often see that it's the movement side of the equation that is lacking as we generally set a calorie deficit on paper, which is around 500 kcal below their maintenance. If they hit their movement targets, then they generally make progress in terms of visible body composition changes and average weight loss. If we only measured weight on the scales once a week, like a lot of the big weight-loss groups do, then our information is severely restricted and therefore our actions may be ineffective.

There is another element I want to make sure that you are aware of. This is the body composition change that comes from a leaner lifestyle. Many of my female clients experience this to varying degrees and it can become a really difficult situation if you aren't monitoring your changes.

45. BODY COMPOSITION VS BODY WEIGHT

Body composition changes occur when you change the percentage of fat and muscle in your body. Your weight on the scales is actually your mass; this mass is made up of water, bone, fat, muscle and vital organs. As discussed earlier, water levels can change quickly, as can glycogen stored in the muscle. You can't really change your bone or vital organ weight without a chainsaw and a scalpel, so when fat and muscle shift their percentages in the body, it's quite noticeable.

Think of this scenario – a person who is relatively sedentary and overweight suddenly decides that they want to get in shape and lose some weight. They start training with weights and moving more, which stimulates muscle building. At the same time, they restrict their calorie intake, eat healthier, eat more protein and less dietary fat. This stimulates fat burning as a fuel from the deficit. In the next 3 months they lose 4 kg of body fat and gain 1–2 kg of muscle. We know that muscle holds glycogen, which in turn can hold up to four times its weight in water.

The resulting loss in fat and gain in muscle might be shown on the scales as a very small, *if at all*, variance in body weight. This can be incredibly disheartening for the client until we look at the progress photos that I always recommend clients take of themselves every few weeks. This would show a clear change and goes a long way to the client regaining confidence and motivation.

I had first-hand experience of this when one year I dieted for the South Coast Championship and my weight started at 92 kg. Twelve weeks later it was still 92 kg. Quite annoying but I was improving day by day. Even so, I also had a weight making consideration to think about and I needed to be 90 kg to make the light heavyweights. In the last few weeks, under some guidance from my closest friend Paul Scarborough (himself an expert prep coach), I dropped into the 89.9 kg bracket for show day.

Ironically, I ended up winning the overall best bodybuilder for that show, so it wouldn't have mattered if I had made the weight or not, and I actually looked better at 92 kg, so by dropping the weight I may have actually put myself at risk of not winning. An important lesson that weight on the scales is never the true indicator of your progression or how good you look.

Case Study – Hannah's transformation

Hannah is a long-term client of mine who has seen tremendous change in her body composition. She is a vet and so the option for severe low carbing, resulting in lack of concentration, is out, as people tend to get upset if you have an accident with their animal. We have been working on a long-term strategy to increase output and focus on slow deficits, which allows Hannah to still keep up her busy social life and make steady progress.

Over the course of a year, Hannah went from 71 kg to 67 kg. Hardly a newsworthy weight drop over the time when just looking at the numbers, but when looking at her progress pictures, the story was very clear. There was a visible drop in body fat and increase in muscle over the period, but what's more relevant is that her bodyweight now stays around the 67 kg mark, even if she has a week or two off for holidays where she can't really track or monitor anything.

This is relevant because the body has a set point where it is happy with the amount of body fat it prefers to keep at a 'normal' level. This is called the Lipostat. Like a thermostat in a room but for body fat.

If you can train the body to reduce lipostat setting, then you can essentially maintain a lower body fat level without maintaining a super strict diet all of the time. In essence, the body will work to maintain the lower level and adjust hunger and energy output levels accordingly. This is the leaner lifestyle in action.

More interestingly, Hannah has only dropped her average calorie intake from 1,700 to 1,600 per day over the year. You don't need massive calorie drops to make progress, just consistency in what you do, and Hannah is one of the most consistent clients I've worked with.

Hannah has also increased her exercise level and as well as training with weights 4–5 times a week she does a weekly boxing session and takes part in the Krav Maga classes that the gym hosts.

Now I know what you're thinking, that she's increased her energy output levels, which is why she's so much leaner. While she has increased her output slightly, Hannah has actually traded in her previous routines of boring cardio on the treadmill for more active and fun activities to burn calories.

This makes so much more sense. If you enjoy something, you'll work harder at it and get more out of it. Same as how your diet must fit your lifestyle, your exercise must fit your interests.

You can see Hannah's transformation photos and her stats including calories in, bodyweight steps and estimated cardio at www.bkmnutrition.com/hannah

46. FAT BURNERS

"According to the Global Weight Loss and Weight Management Market report, the Weight Loss and Weight Management Market accounted a value of $168.95 billion in 2016 and is projected to reach a value $278.95 billion at the end of 2023"

Reuters 16th Jan 2018.

Alongside the diet gurus and weight-loss programmes that exist, you also have the surgeons performing stomach stapling and gastric bypasses to help or force people to lose weight.

In addition to all of this you've got the fat-burner market. The market for fat burners is expected to grow by 7% between 2018 and 2023 according to Mordor Intelligence, so there's certainly no downturn in the number of people looking for a quick fix for their weight-loss issues.

Do fat burners really work though? They must do to some degree if people keep buying them, surely?

Fat burners cover a broad range of supplements and vary in their effectiveness and strength due to the multitude of different compounds that are in them. This topic is so vast that I could write almost a whole other book on it. However, it would be incredibly boring, so here's a brief overview of the key points that you need to know.

1. **Fat Burners won't work without a calorie deficit**
   This pretty much says it all. No matter the strength of the product, body fat will only be used as fuel by the body in a calorie deficit and certainly no product exists that will 'melt fat' off you in four weeks like some claim. The basic rules of thermogenesis apply, and you must eat less than you expend.

2. **Most of the strongest ones are stimulants**
   You'll most likely see caffeine as part of the make-up of the vast majority of sports-based fat burners. Caffeine acts an agent to facilitate fat loss by increasing adrenaline, which in turn acts on a hormone called hormone-sensitive lipase (HSL).

   This causes a cascade, which ultimately results in the release of free fatty acids (FFA) from body fat to be used as fuel. This sounds really cool and like a slam dunk for using stimulants as a fat burner, but the issue is that even if the FFAs are released, there's zero guarantee that they will make it into the actual muscle cells for use as fuel during exercise. It's more likely that they'll be released into the blood, float about for a bit and then the majority will be re-esterified (turned back into body fat) later on.

This is because ...

3. **Fat requires a transporter to get into cells to be burned as fuel**
   A transporter is like a truck that carries a cargo to a destination. In this case the cargo is fat, and the truck is an amino acid called carnitine. The first problem is most people only have a very limited amount of carnitine in their body. The next problem is that if you're working out really hard carnitine may be used as a buffer for exercise rather than transporting fat into cells. What that means is the body uses it to help you continue exercising rather than thinking about your fat-loss efforts. An example would be when your legs are burning from an intense spin class, carnitine may be used to help you keep pedalling by reducing muscle soreness from lactic acid.

   Even worse if you are a quite fit person anyway, you'll use something called IMTAGs (intra-muscular triacylglycerides) to burn as a fat fuel source because they are already in the muscle, stored similarly to how the body stores glycogen for quick use.

   If you're a very overweight person then you'll burn a higher percentage of body fat for fuel in exercise. This is because you don't possess enough of the enzymes in the muscles to break down and use IMTAGs for fuel. The more you exercise, the less you'll use body fat and the more you'll use IMTAGs as you start to produce more of these enzymes.

Life is cruel like that.

4. **Carnitine in most supplements is worthless**
   I bet you read number 3 and thought, "awesome, I'll overdose some carnitine." Unfortunately, most of the carnitine sold as a fat loss aid is pretty rubbish in helping with fat loss. If you are going down the supplemental carnitine route you want a specific form called L-Carnitine-L-Tartrate. Most other L Carnitine supplements are worthless in my opinion, and they are included in a lot of supplements as a lazy and cheap addition, also, nowhere near the actual dose used in clinical trials to be effective.

5. **Many fat burners use diuretics**
   What's the measure of success? For most people it's weight loss. So, when you start to see the scales going down, and if you haven't read this book, you'll immediately think your fat burner is working. If it's mostly water though, those results mean zero in terms of fat loss. Look out for supplements containing dandelion (taraxacum), uva ursi, celery seed or olive leaf as a principal ingredient, and you'll know there's a diuretic angle being played. This practice is deceptive unless of course it's part of an actual diuretic supplement, which really should only be used under very specific circumstances.

6. **The effects of fat burners will always be temporary**
   This is the main reason why I don't recommend them for clients as the effects will only really last while you are using them. This is fine if you know this and accept it for use preparing for a special event like a holiday or competition. However, they should never be used as a 'kick start' for your diet as you'll rebound on your progress and regain weight once you stop. This can be depressing and demotivating, even if you are expecting it, and can interfere with your overall progress.

7. **Some companies add fat to fat burners to help you burn fat**
   This is so stupidly counterproductive that I can't even begin to form a phrase to describe the idiocy of it. It's something that does exist though. Remember when I said that fat requires a transporter to get into cells to be burned as fuel? Well there's one type of fat that doesn't and that's MCTs or medium chain triglycerides. These have a structure that allows them to pass through the cell membrane and be used quickly for fuel in the cell. Sounds great? Until you realise that MCTs don't come from body fat.

   They are included in fat-loss supplements so that they can claim that the supplement gets into your system and starts burning fat almost immediately. It's the MCTs not the body fat that get burned, and this presents even more of a block for FFAs from your body fat making it into the cells to be burned as fuel. Also, supplements that add ketone salts, such as BHB (beta-hydroxybutyrate), look to put your body into an artificially created state of ketosis because the salts will cause ketones to rise in the blood.

There's actually no evidence at the time of writing that shows that keto salts help with fat loss where there wasn't already a calorie deficit in place. It's still an emerging area of research, but one critical factor that has been seen is that keto salts actually reduce the power output in workouts because they restrict the use of glycogen as a fuel, which isn't good if you like benching or squatting heavy, or doing lots of HIT work (high-intensity training). My advice would be to stay away from these types of supplements completely.

As a parting note on this topic, there is some research showing a beneficial effect of including MCTs as a higher component of your diet than normal dietary fat, such as animal fats, in terms of higher fat oxidation (burning). So, if you are able to swap out some fats for coconut oil or butter, which both contain a higher percentage of MCT in their make-up, this *may* help you a little bit in your diet targets. I'd suggest that sticking to a calorie deficit as your first target would be the best course of action though before overcomplicating with macro variations.

Side note

You may have heard or been told at some point to put butter or coconut oil in your coffee to give you an energy boost. This so-called 'bulletproof coffee' came about due to the MCT content of the two fat sources. I'll be honest, I've had coffee with coconut oil in when I used to do early morning kick-boxing sessions before my gym opened. I did get a boost of energy, but I'd not do it now given what I know about nutrition. I'd most likely have a small carb snack and a caffeine-based pre-workout drink.

As a conclusion to this chapter and section it's very important to note that everything we have discussed always comes back to a calorie deficit as the main driver of fat loss in the body. Fat burners may give you some extra focus in the gym and help you train a bit harder, but you've still got to get into a deficit.

There are so many people and businesses trying to get your money to sell you a dream of a tighter waistline, or to get into that little black dress, that they will say pretty much anything within the Advertising Standards Authority or Facebook ads rules to do it.

There will be a lot of scientific-sounding phrases thrown at you, never more so than on supplements that will list the chemical or scientific names for a product rather than just saying what they are in common language. Things like ascorbic acid (vitamin C) or white willow bark (the base form of aspirin) are regularly thrown about in supplements to make something sound complicated when it's really not.

Weight-loss companies will get you to follow their formulas or set diet systems to get you to lose weight, but all the time they are building up your reliance on their system or supplements when really all they have done is put you in a calorie deficit. The problem is, of course, that we as humans don't like endless imprisonment in our routines. If you never take a holiday from your work or always work weekends, then you will burn out. Most diet plans or systems don't really account for this, even the big ones with their made up codes for classification of foods with the same calories as 'good' or 'bad' for the diet. It's normally these breaks from routine that light the fuse leading to a Prison Break from a diet and so we have to account for the breaks in our overall plan.

We also need to remember that the human body is not a closed system. It is not a computer doing the same programmed routines every time with the same outcome. Numerous factors affect our biology and so measuring just one factor such as a once-weekly weigh-in is completely irrelevant to overall progress.

If we are to be successful in living a leaner lifestyle and as a result losing body fat for the long term, then we need to have a plan that reflects the various physical, social, psychological and environmental influences that affect us.

Living a leaner lifestyle is not something you do for twelve weeks to lose a bit of weight for a holiday, that's a results, or goal-driven activity, and it reflects the mindset that "I am an overweight person trying to lose XX kg."

What we want to do to be successful is think, "I want to live life like a XX kg person, so how can I change my lifestyle to do this?"

Having a mindset of a leaner person, casting votes every day for that leaner person, will result in that person becoming real.

I want you to stop thinking about the goal and start thinking about the systems that we can put in place to make sure you get there and stay there. Then the rest will be easy.

SECTION 2

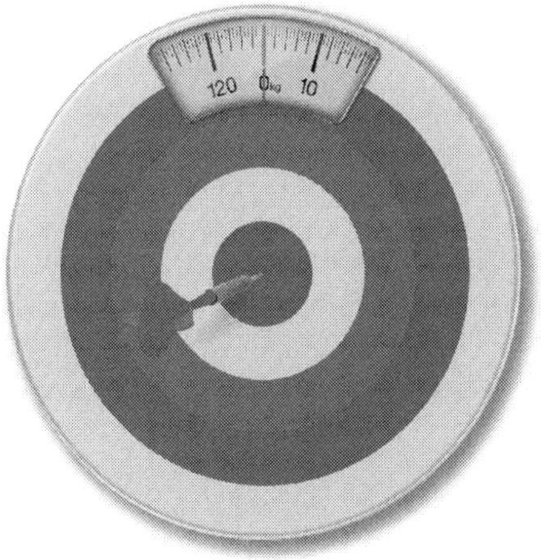

48. THE FOREST OF ABBREVIATIONS

Before we get into the nuts and bolts of your diet plan there are some concepts that you need to be aware of so that you can talk in nutritionists' lingo. I've bunched them all here so that you can quick reference them if you need to.

RMR

TEF, NEAT

EAT, EER

These are the main abbreviations that nutrition people like to use when discussing diets.

RMR – Resting Metabolic Rate
This is the energy you use every day to survive. If you were in a coma this would be your expenditure to keep your brain, lungs, etc. working so that you stay alive. When working out your calorie intake for weight loss we generally don't want to go below this, but it's not the end of the world if you do occasionally.

TEF – Thermic Effect of Food

The calories that you use every day digesting your food. I've discussed this at length previously, go back and have a re-read if you missed it.

NEAT – Non-Exercise Activity Thermogenesis

I've touched on this briefly. This is the next biggest energy consumer in most people and it's the energy you expend moving around in your daily life. When you fidget, walk to the toilet, scroll through Facebook, walk around the supermarket, that's all NEAT. If you are a postman your NEAT would normally be higher than a sedentary nine-to-five office worker, and this will have an effect on how many calories you can eat in the day.

EAT – Exercise Activity Thermogenesis

As you may have guessed, this is all the energy you expend exercising. This is generally anything that gets your heart rate above normal for a period of time. People think that this is the most important thing to focus on when losing weight. Actually, for most people it will not be higher than 20–25% of their daily output and NEAT will be the main consumer, so remember that when you're sitting on your couch daydreaming about the gym.

EER – Energy Expenditure Rate

Also called TDEE – Total Daily Energy Expenditure. This is basically all the four elements above added together to give you an idea of your maintenance calories. This is the number of calories you can eat or drink to remain exactly where you are, no fat loss or gain. Notice I said *fat* loss or gain. It's perfectly possible to gain muscle in a calorie deficit or maintenance situation and that's important to remember when we look at long-term body composition improvements.

49. CICO – THE NAUGHTY MONKEY

CICO is calories in, calories out. It's the thing, if you follow any nutrition educators, that you'll see debated to high heaven with those who are not as well educated. This is the fundamental argument based on the laws of thermodynamics. Energy cannot be created or destroyed, and it can't just disappear. Energy is contained in food and when we eat, we obtain a certain amount of energy from the meal, which we use to fuel the body or store as energy. Some is also lost in heat.

Thermodynamics is a boring subject if you aren't a nerd like me, so let's just say that the food calories you put into your body must be burned off in activity as part of your TDEE or it will become stored. This will be either as glycogen in the muscles and liver or as adipose tissue, which is body fat. Some fat also ends up in the muscle as IMTAGs, which I discussed in the final chapter of Section 1.

The reason why CICO is a naughty monkey is that it rarely plays fair. You never really know what your calories-out are, even if you have a Fitbit or similar device. You can only really guess. You can't tell exactly what your calories-in are either. This is due to something called entropy, which is the energy lost in the form of heat generated by from the process of converting energy. Sometimes you won't fully gain all the energy in a food, and sometimes you'll get a more efficient digestion. This can be based on a number of factors including enzyme activity. Enzymes help break down foods and facilitate reactions in the body. Gut health is also vital for digestion efficiency.

With CICO you're always giving it your best guess, which is why it's a good idea to hedge your bets and if you're trying to lose body fat make sure you have a decent deficit amount on paper that allows for any contingency.

50. ALL FOODS ARE NOT EQUAL; SOME ARE MORE EQUAL THAN OTHERS

You may have heard people argue over macro-based diets. These are diets that are based on a certain amount of protein, carbs and fats (macros) in a diet to give a calorie amount for fat loss or muscle gain. Why macro diets come under attack is that it will simply say, "eat X g of protein, X g of carbs, X g of fats in a day", without reference or guidance to many of the topics I've discussed here.

There is good research showing that processed foods are easier to get calories out of than unprocessed. For example, a study done on peanut butter vs the equivalent weight and calories of peanuts, showed that more calories were gained from the peanut butter. This is logical as the peanuts have already been broken down to an extent by the process of crushing them into peanut butter; in essence they are pre-digested. The same is true of cooking food or mashing, mincing and juicing. All these processes change the state of the food in some way from its natural state and make the calories more accessible.

Therefore, a meal of brown rice cakes and peanut butter will yield more usable calories than boiled brown rice and peanuts even though on paper they may have the same calorie value.

Another consideration is that, a processed vs unprocessed diet comparison study discovered that people eating the processed diet tended to overeat more than the unprocessed. This is likely due to the reduction in fibre and perhaps a drop in TEF. Coupled with a faster digestion this could mean the people did not feel full up for as long and so snacked or ate more at the next meal.

This is an important consideration when you're thinking about what to have in your diet. Although calories are a serious factor and should be the first priority, the type of food you are eating should also be on your list of considerations. If you decide to make up your diet from mainly processed food, then you may find your hunger returns faster and the diet is harder to stick to.

While calories are the ultimate determinant of success on a diet, where you get those calories from can determine how easy it is to stay within the lines.

51. THE GOOD, THE BAD AND THE HEALTHY

A concept that you must get your head around is that there is no inherently good or bad food. It's probably been drilled into you from an early age that certain foods are 'treats' or 'naughty' and some foods are 'healthy'. Living a leaner lifestyle means that we rise above that level of distinction and start being a bit more like Tivor – logical, reasoned and calm – in our view of nutrition.

For example, avocados are always touted as being a healthy food, and why not? They contain antioxidants and vitamins, some fibre and unsaturated fats. Plus, they are green and green means healthy, or at least it does to some weird diets that classify on colour. I'm not disputing that avocados are a good food to include in your diet if you like them. However, the thing you need to consider is that they contain a bucket load of calories – around 140 per half an average avocado.

A large number of my clients swear blind at our first consultation that they are eating all healthy foods and no rubbish but cannot lose weight. When I look at their diet recall, a three-day journal I ask them to keep, they are having loads of healthy foods that are loaded with calories, and this is causing them to gain fat.

The usual suspects here are

- Avocados
- Coconut Oil
- Olive Oil
- Nuts
- Pasta
- Salmon
- Smoothies
- Cheese

There are others of course but these are the ones that pop up repeatedly and are all very calorie dense in nature compared to their volume or the space they occupy on the plate. I have included pasta on this list both for its calorific value, but also as certain weight-loss programmes have classed it as a 'Free Food' and you end up with women piling up their plates with pasta, which actually contains 322 kcal per 100 g.

Did you also notice that a lot of these are also 'healthy fat' containing foods? There's a good number of gurus advising that loads of healthy fats will somehow ramp up your metabolism and prevent you gaining body fat. See Chapter 42 on big fat lies if you missed it for the reasons why this isn't the case.

Like I said previously, I have no issue with these foods, and I eat all of them myself apart from cheese. *I hate cheese! Yuck.* However, you must pay attention to the potential for overeating when adding these foods to a meal and account for them in your calorie intake.

Thankfully, there are a few really good apps that can help you with this.

Also, make sure that you add some traditionally bad foods into your diet. Living a leaner lifestyle doesn't mean you live like a Spartan and never enjoy a burger or pizza; it's food for the heart and soul that you occasionally need in order to relax and unwind. Celery sticks just don't do it for me when I'm watching a movie. Popcorn and some pick and mix are fine if accounted for in your calorie plan and it's not going to make you ill eating them. I say this as I had a client once account for 2,000 calories on his higher calorie day with pick and mix. He was not in a good way that evening.

52. JUDGEMENT DAY – RISE OF THE MACHINES

Many people nowadays have Fitbits or other monitoring devices that track their steps and calories, etc. I myself have an Apple watch because I'm a serial Apple cultist and all my stuff is Apple. They are a great motivational tool to help increase your activity and log your progress in living a leaner lifestyle, but always be vigilant when using them.

A study done on a range of wrist-worn devices highlighted that there can be as much as a 500 kcal variation in these devices when calculating daily expenditure of calories. I've had a few clients tell me that they have not lost weight despite being in a deficit after they've logged their activity from their watch and eaten to that amount. The same is true on apps such as *MyFitnessPal*, which gives you an estimate of your activity from training and then tells you how much food you can eat to balance it.

My advice is not to trust these readings at all. Although there are some very accurate, new devices coming out, and may already be out by the time you read this book, the only really accurate measure of activity is a device called an *ActiHeart*, which costs around £10,000 and straps to your chest measuring any acceleration of your heartbeat.

Unless you've got £10,000 to randomly drop on one of these devices, then you should just use your device as a measure of average activity. For example, if you track your activity and steps for a few weeks and log it against your calorie intake, then you will get a trend of activity so you can see if you have been more or less active and how that has affected your weight average.

Remember that if you track trends then over time the error margin reduces as you are tracking a trend and not a value. If the value is always 400 kcal out, and you increase by 400 kcal, then you'll still be 400 kcal off the real figure, but you'll have increased your activity, which can be measured.

We are always looking at average behaviour because humans are not a closed system like a desktop computer and many outside variables affect our results. Tracking trends and not focussing on specific values can be a very helpful process.

SECTION 3

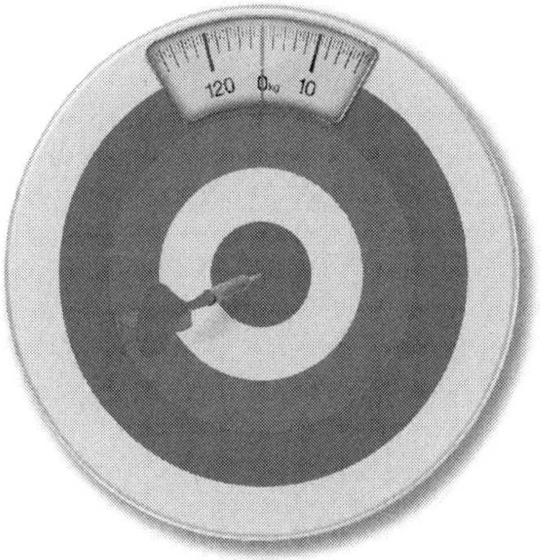

53. LET'S GET DOWN TO BUSINESS

By now you should be fully armed with all the information you need to identify rogue diet gurus and some of the complete idiocy that people come out with for their diets. You should never fall into any of their get-slim-quick schemes again.

Now it's time to start building your bulletproof plan that's tailored to your own lifestyle and routines.

In this section I'll show you how to:

- Identify your safe and trigger foods and how to build in safeguards to prevent binges
- Calculate your own calories for weight loss
- Build meals that you like and fit them to your busy day
- Work **with** your brain so that you give your Muncher brain enough treats to keep it at bay and out of your decision making.

- Plan for failure so that if you fall off the wagon you can get straight back on again, easily
- Prepare for big social events so that you can enjoy buffets and birthday cake without stressing about going off the rails
- Build strong habits to change your mindset from being a dieter to a leaner lifestyle activist
- Remove self-sabotaging processes from your life to stop you being your own worst enemy

I can confidently say that if you apply the rules and processes I have laid out in the next few chapters, you will absolutely not feel as if you are dieting ever again. The most common feedback we get from the Target Lean programme is that the members just feel like they are eating what they like and losing weight.

I talked previously about the three pressure points of confusion, prison and frustration. To counter these negative factors, I work with a three-pronged solution to these issues and they are:

Clarity

Choice

Consistency

The three Cs are interlinked in a similar way to how the three pressure points are and excelling on one will enhance the other. When you have developed strong elements of each factor your progress will be unstoppable, and you'll understand exactly why you failed before and will never make that mistake again.

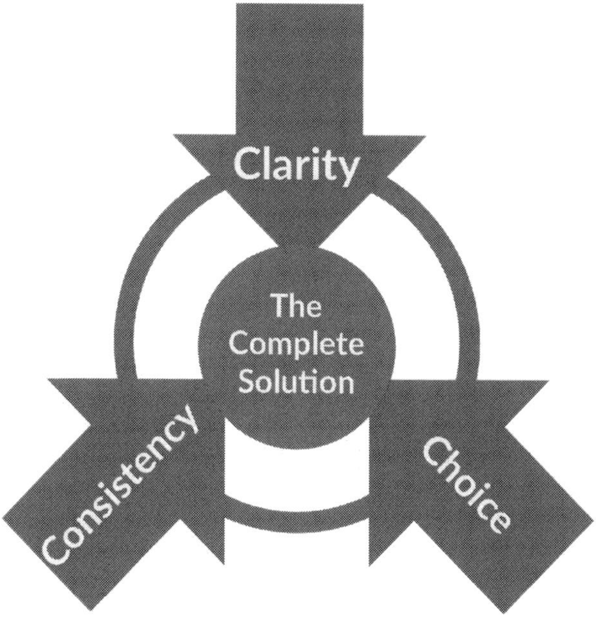

Clarity

I've highlighted throughout this book that confusion about nutrition is one of the main drivers of behaviour that you later find out is 'the wrong thing to do'. Fad diets, fasted cardio, detoxes and other weird things people do come about because people do not know what the best way is to lose weight. This whole book is about giving you clarity and wiping away the confusion.

Having the knowledge about why things work and when to use certain techniques means you will always have a clarity of purpose and know exactly the strategies you need to implement in order to continue progressing.

The more consistent that you are in your actions, leading to positive results, the clearer you will become in your decision making. The key principle for losing body fat is to create a calorie deficit. If you do not know how to do that then you will never have success on your diet. You must have clarity and no confusion so that you have clear direction based in knowledge.

Choice

The prison creates restriction and takes choice away from you. It's their rules and you are just here for the ride. Most people fall off, some quite badly. They are not invested in the diet they follow because they don't understand it; they have no clarity, so they have no choice.

You *can* choose exactly what you eat, *when* you eat it and *what* systems you employ.

Some of the techniques in this book may not be relevant to you right away, maybe they never will. However, knowing them will mean that when a problem comes up that you need to deal with, you will have that option to choose from. Some situations will have many potential solutions; choice gives you the option to pick the one that you prefer the most, meaning that you're more likely to follow it. The more you make consistent positive choices the clearer you become on which ones are the right ones for your progress.

Consistency

This is the crucial aspect of any successful diet programme; follow a diet for one day and nothing happens, follow it for three to four weeks and you can see dramatic changes. Only having clarity and choice in place means that you can be consistent. It doesn't mean that you do the same thing every day, but you cast consistent votes for a leaner lifestyle. The more you vote for the life you want, the more you will become that life. Clarity and choice allow you to continue to make votes for the better, and consistent votes make clarity more defined and choice easier to do.

Key Point

It's very important that you don't try to be 100% perfect with your diet all of the time. Trying to be perfect never works. Some situations just don't allow it. However, if you can hit a consistent 80% or more, you will always make progress.

Aiming for 100% forces you to dwell on your mistakes. Having clarity means that you know that things won't be perfect all of the time and you make a choice to be OK with that and focus on being consistent with the things that you can control.

54. 'EATING WHAT YOU LIKE' AND 'EATING WHAT YOU LIKE'

I just want to make this clear before we start. When I say you can eat whatever foods that you like, I do mean that you can incorporate any food that you like eating into your diet.

What I don't mean is that you can face-plant cake every day until it's oozing out of your ears and hope to lose weight. If I had that secret this book would be £10,000 an edition and I'd be driving a different Ferrari every week.

You can eat cake every day for sure, but that will mean you won't be as full up and you'll have to be in better control of your snacking instinct and tolerate more hunger.

What I want to emphasise again is that there is no good or bad food on this diet. For me, if I eat Hobnobs I generally swallow a whole packet, so I don't eat them often. I can, however, have a few biscuits and not want anymore. With this in mind, let's get into planning your LEAN Matrix.

55. THE LEAN MATRIX

The major failure of most diets is that they don't address the foods that are specific to you as a person and your Muncher as a snacking driver.

A useful process I undertake with new clients is to give them the LEAN Matrix planner.

How it works is as follows.

I want you to draw one big square on a piece of paper and then divide it into four equal squares. This represents the four sectors for food in your life and is based on the amount of impulse control you have over a food and then the reward response that you get from that food. You need to plot the foods you eat in your daily life into these squares.

The left-hand, vertical line of the graph is Impulse Control and the bottom line is Reward Response. Think of it like an X and Y axis where the further up or right you go the more that axis has strength. Here is a diagram to help you.

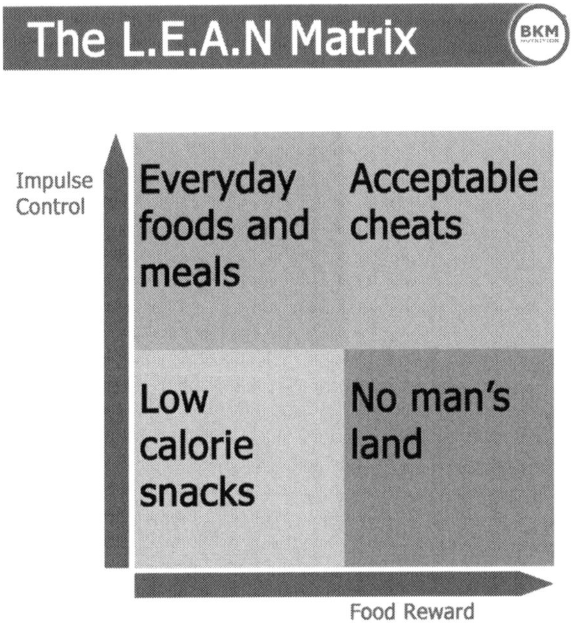

The sections should be labelled like this:

Top Left – Everyday foods and meals

This is food that you have high impulse control over and gives you a small to moderate food reward response. For me, this would be chicken and rice with spinach. It's a meal I like, and I eat every day, but once I've eaten a decent amount, I don't want any more.

Bottom Left – Low calorie snacks

These are foods that you have lower impulse control over but carry a low reward response, for example, a fruit bowl in an office reception that has green apples in it may fall into this area as you are likely to pick up and eat an apple (low impulse control) but unlikely to binge on all the apples in the bowl. One is enough. Also, biscuits from the tin at coffee time where you only eat one, a few crisps from a colleague's packet or your own packet that doesn't cause a binge. These should form your low-impact snacks in between your main meals drawn from the top left. I generally have fruit or Snack a Jacks in this area.

Top Right – Acceptable cheats

I know the word cheat implies a bad food but it's something that people can understand as a term, so I keep it in. Indulgences sounds a bit posh for me, even though I went to a posh grammar school. With high reward response you get a lot of pleasure from these foods, but with high impulse control you can eat some and then are satisfied. These are foods/meals that you can add in as an 'off the plan' meal to have with friends or relaxing but don't cause a binge.

For example, I class Nando's in this area for me. Nando's is a higher calorie meal than I'd eat normally, and I only have it occasionally, but if I eat it, I don't immediately want another, and I wouldn't eat it to bursting. It satisfies me for a few hours. These should be meals for you that do the same, they can be meals or foods you like as a treat, can be a beer if you enjoy a beer watching the TV like I do as long as that beer doesn't lead to a snack attack of crisps or similar, which is uncontrollable and plunges you into ...

Key Point

Apps like *MyFitnessPal* or *Eat This Much* can help you determine the calorie values of many popular restaurants. I also have a guide to eating out that you can download free from my website at www.bkmnutrition.com/eatingout. Remember that, within your calorie allowance, we can factor in pretty much any food you want to eat. I'll show you how to calculate your calories for fat loss in the following chapters.

Bottom Right – No man's land

This is really where you don't want to be. These are the foods that plunge you into an uncontrollable frenzy of food destruction. Low impulse control and high reward response mean that your brain wants more of these foods and you are powerless to resist. For a lot of people this will be ice cream, pizza, biscuits, doughnuts, beer, Haribos – all high calorie-laden foods. Funny that none of the high calorie healthy foods that I listed earlier feature here. I've never had a client have uncontrollable urges for avocados. Well, not for eating anyway.

It's important for you to be honest with yourself and to put the foods in here that really trigger you. We want to work with your brain and that means limiting your exposure to things that will really challenge you.

Key Point

Many people overthink this section. It's the foods or meals that trigger you; that could be individual food items or combinations of foods. For example, potatoes aren't really a trigger food, but chips might be. Steak on on its own may not be a trigger food but steak and chips might be. Normally, you'll find that trigger foods are highly processed foods that you purchase ready to eat. Food companies have people sitting in rooms investigating the perfect combinations of salt, sugar and fat to keep you eating them until you can't eat any more. These are the foods that are triggers for most people. Being in no man's land does *not* mean that you should never eat these foods, but it allows us to be more mindful of our consumption when they are in our hands.

No matter how hard you try you will sometimes find yourself deep in no man's land viciously hoovering up some pick and mix before you realise what you are doing. That's OK and it happens to everyone, but having this matrix in place will allow you to quickly navigate out of the minefield and into greener pastures.

Remember, *no* planning and *no* processes mean you will repeatedly be firefighting your problems. Problems will always come up; having the right plans in place and the processes to implement them means that problems will remain small. You will face lots of challenges at first but keeping the three Cs in mind will help you immensely in combatting them.

You can download a free copy of the LEAN Matrix at www.bkmnutrition.com/lean-matrix. There is also a helpful video to explain this topic and guide you through. If you're still stuck, feel free to post in my Facebook group – Target Lean Lifestyle, and I'll be happy to help.

I cannot stress how important this exercise is so before you read on, draw up your LEAN Matrix and plot your foods on it. Writing is better than doing it on a computer as the brain remembers more of what you write than what you type.

Activity

1. Get a piece of paper
2. Plot your LEAN Matrix
3. Add all your foods in and be honest
4. Email me if you have any questions
5. Post a pic of your LEAN Matrix on Instagram #LEANMATRIX and tag me in it @ tomblackman_nutrition and I'll send you a free recipe book as a reward. Make sure you check your DMs and don't block me ☺

56. THE C.A.L.O.R.I.E. SYSTEM

Without a doubt this system has been the simplest way to allow the people I work with to take control of their own diets and lifestyle.

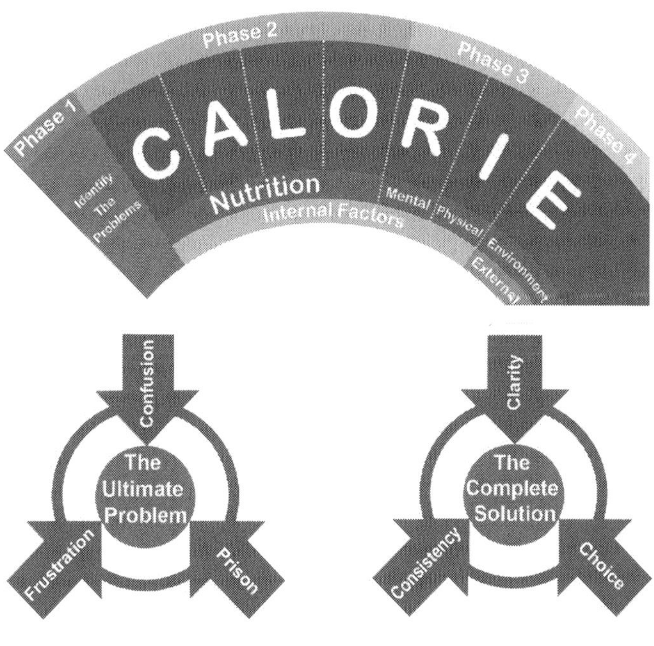

I have used this framework with over 200 private clients at the time of writing this book and it's incredibly effective at producing long-term results. You can use this for both weight loss and muscle gain, but for the purposes of this book, we will of course be focussing on weight or fat loss.

C.A.L.O.R.I.E. is made up of:

- **C**alculate
- **A**llocate
- **L**ist
- **O**rganise
- **R**outine
- **I**ncrease activity
- **E**valuate

The C.A.L.O.R.I.E. system is a seven-step process and it's important to understand that each step is a link in a chain. If one link is weak then your results will be less dramatic or even non-existent. If you follow this process exactly then you will always see improvements in your fat-loss efforts. If you have reached a sticking point, it's because one of the steps is not being done correctly.

Calculate your calories for weight loss

Remember that calories are the ultimate determinant for weight loss, so before we get into macros, or even 'If it fits your macros', we need to know how many calories you need to be eating for fat loss.

This can be a bit of a minefield because every person is different in their daily routines. As a nutritionist I have to take into account not only their biological metrics such as height, weight, age, etc. but also their daily activity, what their job is and how that affects their calorie needs. If they are a more muscled person, that will also affect things slightly.

For you though, you only need to think about your own environment and therefore these values will change only slightly.

There are a number of ways that you can calculate your own calories.

As we go through, I will use an example of a 100 kg male to illustrate the calculations. You'll find it much easier to use kg in calculations, and most modern calculators will use metric measurements such as kilograms, metres and litres.

1. **Use a really basic rule of thumb – not recommended**
   Sometimes (all the time) when I meet new people and they find out I'm a nutritionist they immediately ask me what to eat to lose weight, and of course I explain it's to do with calories, and I use a rough rule of thumb to work out their calorie needs. This is based on the accepted rough calculation that males burn approximately 1.0 kcal per kg of bodyweight per hour, and females burn slightly less at 0.9 kcal per kg of bodyweight.

   This means that you can work out a rough estimate of your calories for the day by multiplying your bodyweight by 24 if you are male, or 22 if you are female.

This will give you a very rough estimate and it's worth noting that if you are very overweight then this figure will most likely be skewed.

For our 100 kg male the calculation would go like this: 100 kg x 24 = 2,400 kcal per day.

Personally, I'd stay away from this as an accurate means of calculating your calories for the day, as the margin for error could be quite high, especially if you are somewhat overweight. It's more for a basic check that I'd use to look at a person's calorie intake at a first glance.

I would never use this method to actually construct a client's diet plan, especially as I pay big bucks for an advanced nutrition software programme that uses a variety of metrics to make it more exact.

What if you don't have that programme though?

2. **Use an online calculator – recommended**
   Lucky for you, I've actually made my own calculator that is free to use on my website. Simply go to www.bkmnutrition.com/calculator and you can access the free calculator I've made that uses all the advanced metrics such as adding in variables for your job and exercise activity.

   It will also give you a guideline for the amounts of protein, carbs and fats to aim for in your daily intake, if you prefer to do your tracking that way.

> Of course, there are other calculators on the web that you can use, and they all use slightly different variables and formulas to get a number. Don't get too concerned if you get results that are varied in their number, as different formulas will give slightly different outcomes. A variance of about 10–15% is fine.
>
> A word of advice here, don't overcomplicate the variables too much. A lot of calculators will ask for things like days you train, how long, what muscle groups, etc. This is totally overcomplicating things for the sake of – most likely – selling you their programme or diet sheet that's tailored to your DNA or something equally ludicrous.

The idea with calculating your calories is just to *get a starting point*.

You need a peg in the sand to start and you can always adjust as you go.

Allocate these calories over meals

Now that we have our figure for calories, we need to do something with them, and this step involves splitting the calories into meal sizes.

You'll need to have an idea of your daily routine and what will work best for you. For example, I prefer three to four bigger meals in the day over five to six smaller meals. It's also important that you allocate some of the calories to snacks and not just decide you'll only eat at mealtimes as this almost never happens, and you'll end up overeating (cheating).

Let's look at two options: the bigger less frequent meals and the smaller more frequent meals.

I will use my 2,400 figure from my 100 kg male.

3 meals a day plus 1 snack 'meal' block = 4 blocks

2,400 kcal ÷ 4 blocks = 4 x 600 kcal meals

Breakfast	–	600 kcal
Lunch	–	600 kcal
Dinner	–	600 kcal
Snacks	–	600 kcal total for the day

5 meals a day plus 1 snack 'meal' block = 6 blocks

2,400 ÷ 6 = 400 kcal meals

Breakfast	–	400 kcal
Mid-morning	–	400 kcal
Lunch	–	400 kcal
Mid-afternoon	–	400 kcal
Dinner	–	400 kcal
Snacks	–	400 kcal total for the day

It's really important to be honest with yourself in your assessment here as this process sets the foundation of your meals. As an idea of meal sizes, anything under 150 kcal I would class as a snack. You won't get much for your money with 150 kcal, so don't think you'll be eating 8 'meals' of 150 kcal. That will be a day of snacks.

There's nothing wrong with this of course but for meals you really want 250 kcal and upwards.

By the way, there is nothing stopping you bunching meals together for a bigger meal if you want to. We will cover this later; you just need a template to work from for now.

List foods that you like to eat

This bit is easy. Look back at the LEAN Matrix that you did. These are all the foods that you add into your regular meals apart from the no man's land foods.

Mainly you want to make up your meals from the two left-hand columns – everyday food and low-impact snacks. Keep acceptable cheats for your social days or when you need to have a bit of a splurge. Limiting your meals to everyday foods and low-impact snacks gives you the power of choice and also allows you to gain consistency by staying within your calorie limits while eating foods that you like.

Organise the foods into the meal blocks

Now you need to take those foods and make up some meals.

For me it might look like this:

Breakfast – Eggs and bagels with some fruit.
Lunch – Beef chilli and rice with salad.
Dinner – Salmon and potato with veg.
Snacks – Protein shake and fruit in the day.

To get the calories and food amounts right you'll need to use an app that gives you food values and calories. My default that I use is *MyFitnessPal* as it's pretty user-friendly and simple for most people to use. If you want to watch a video on setting up and using the programme go to www.bkmnutrition.com/myfitnesspal where there is a tutorial video waiting for you.

What I suggest is that you add the foods that would be in the meal then work with the gram measurements until the values fit the calories for the meal. Don't be too finicky about getting it right to the last calorie, a 5–10% variance is OK for the odd meal, but be mindful of the total for the day.

For my 600-kcal breakfast of eggs and bagels:

1 bagel 90 g	=	240 kcal	
4 average eggs	=	300 kcal	(Always have the yolks – they are good for you)
100 g blueberries	=	42 kcal	
Total	=	**582 kcal**	

I'll carry the remaining 18 kcal over to another meal.

Complete this process for all your breakfast and main meal options and snacks until you have a list of two to three different breakfasts, lunches, dinners and snacks. With the snacks, what I generally have is a separate list of snacks and their calorie values and let clients pick from a list until they hit their allowance for the day. You can allocate specific snacks, of course, for the day but it's important to allow yourself the option of swapping out.

I tend to also think of snacks as ways to bump up a meal if you are more hungry, so for example a banana may be in your snacks box but there's nothing stopping you from having it with your lunch as long as the total calories for the day don't exceed your target.

If you would like to download a template for creating your meal plan then go to my website at www.bkmnutrition.com/myfitnesspal.

Routine and habit

I mentioned previously that consistency is one of the key factors for success on a diet and it forms the third arm of the complete solution along with clarity and choice. I'll be covering routine and habit coaching later, but the important thing here is to identify what are your current undesirable habits that you would like to change.

For example, a client I worked with had a routine of coming home and would immediately walk into the kitchen and start snacking on chocolate or other food. It was in her routine to do so and was actually an automated response by her Robot brain and not a trigger by the Muncher brain.

This was obviously not helping her weight-loss efforts and so the solution was to change the routine. We adjusted the sequence to: When she came home, she immediately went to her bedroom and changed clothes. This not only removed the original series of triggers but also reset her environment causing her to break out of her autonomy. The undesirable habit here was snacking when she came home, but you can't just say you'll stop doing it. You need to identify the triggers that cause it and the processes that support it.

To be successful you need to identify the undesirable habits and build barriers to reverting to them. Conversely, you then look at how you can make the desirable habits easier to carry out. A simple example of this is to remove chocolate bars from view in your kitchen and put them at the back of the topmost cupboard shelf. Then put the fruit bowl within your normal walking pattern or field of view. By doing this you are removing the ease of accessibility of chocolate if you have a snack attack and instead placing fruit within easy reach, which is a much lower-calorie option.

Turning your weaknesses into a strength

My sister, Kate, who is a qualified psychologist, used to use a variation of this technique by placing fruit on her desk in the morning rather than leaving it in her bag. Because it was right in front of her, she would eat the fruit rather than getting up and walking across the room to the cake table. In her own words she, "exploited her inherent laziness."

Increase activity

While we have focussed on the calories-in side of the equation in the first half of the C.A.L.O.R.I.E. system, it's very important not to neglect the calories-out side of things.

I've previously discussed NEAT and EAT (see Section 2 for more detailed explanations) and their impact on total daily energy expenditure in the day. As the body starts to recognise that it's in a deficit, it will start to try to slow you down a bit to reduce expenditure of calories. Therefore, it's very important to monitor your activity levels and make a conscious effort to increase them when this happens.

An easy way to do this is to buy a step counter. More people are aware of this and I see many more of my new clients already using their watches to monitor their steps. I ask clients to keep a daily log of this data so that we can recognise when steps, and therefore total body movement, is slowing down. Given that NEAT can be up to 50% of your daily expenditure, a 10% drop in activity can be very significant.

Key point

Our 100 kg man may burn 1,200 calories a day through NEAT activity. If this drops 10% then he's lowered his expenditure by 120 calories. May not seem much but over a week that's 840 calories and over a month that's 3,360 calories. In terms of fat loss, that's potentially 1 lb or 0.5 kg of weight that isn't lost.

Over the year that equates to nearly 6 kg that you may not lose.

Monitoring your steps is therefore vitally important and more often than not when I am assessing a client's progress and we see a slowdown in results, it's generally due to their activity reducing.

Making a purposeful effort to increase activity can have the opposite effect and boost progress. Simple things like taking the stairs and not the lift, or parking your car the furthest away in the car park at the supermarket, are all ways that you can boost activity very simply.

You may be reading this thinking that you don't have many opportunities to increase activity as you work in an office. Using a simple alarm on your watch to buzz you every hour to do a three-minute walk around the building will add a few hundred steps per day to your activity.

Five minutes won't make a difference

One of my clients was an extremely busy mum of four who had incredible demands on her time. Going to the gym wasn't an option, and even time by herself was limited to evenings when she was too tired to do anything. We increased her activity by simply adding five minutes extra distance on her walks to and from school every morning. This equated to just under an hour's extra exercise each week. With calories controlled, this resulted in a body fat drop. It's vitally important to look at what you *can* do and not what you *can't*.

Exercise is associated with lower absence rates at work from illness. As a business owner myself I actively encourage my employees to walk around the building every hour if they've been sedentary for most of that time. There's also a positive benefit from taking a break to give your mind a rest and allow refocussing when you return. I'm actually incredibly bad at taking my own advice though. Therefore, I tend to make up for it when I'm able to by going on walks with my son; normally searching for puddles to jump in.

Case Study – Nathan wanted to get in shape

To illustrate the power of boosting NEAT activity in fat loss, one of my clients, Nathan, came to me for help with getting into shape for his holidays and upcoming stag dos with his friends. Nathan had previously tried to lose weight by restricting carbohydrates and doing extra cardio with mixed results.

When I looked at his activity, he was doing over 25,000 steps a day. The average desk worker does 4,000–6,000 a day, so 25,000 is way above the average. On top of this he was doing cardio and restricting calories. I concluded that he may have been overdoing the activity, which was causing his body a lot of stress.

Due to the high level of activity in his day job as a site supervisor we eliminated any extra cardio and increased his carbohydrates to give him more fuel for his workouts. The result was that his activity level dropped but the reduced stress on his body meant that there was less of a kickback from his metabolism trying to compensate for the huge deficit. He was still in a deficit from his activity, just not an excessive one.

Nathan's daily activity, combined with his food intake, allowed him to get in the best shape of his life. You can see his story at www.bkmnutrition.com/nathan. The purpose of this story is to highlight that to lose weight you don't always need to do a traditional cardio session in the gym to increase activity.

Nathan's activity in his job was enough to facilitate a fat-loss environment and he didn't need to be doing any more cross-trainer or stepper action. By eliminating the cardio, he was able to put more into his weight training and improve his muscle size and shape while cutting body fat. While Nathan's situation is certainly not the normal one for most of my clients, most people can benefit from an increase in their daily activity rather than trying to cram it all in at the gym in sixty minutes.

Evaluate and adjust

What gets measured gets improved. The final stage of the process is to assess your progress and then make the relevant adjustments. The crucial thing to remember here is that you never just use one metric to measure your progress. I generally ask clients to take daily bodyweight readings, weekly progress photos, daily logs of their food intake and a log of their steps in the day. Some clients will also log their cardio and weight training sessions.

While this might seem a lot to do, it allows us to assess at our weekly meetings how things have been affected by any changes we have made.

Most people when dieting only really measure their bodyweight. Worse still, they weigh only once or twice a week. If you have ever been part of a weekly weight-loss group programme, then you'll know the dread of the weigh-in each week.

Your bodyweight fluctuates through the week and you are generally heavier in the evening when most of these meetings are held. Weighing just once a week only gives you a snapshot of your state at that moment.

Remember that the body works on averages; you don't get fat from one day of overeating, and you don't get slim from one day of restriction. Your bodyweight on one day of the week is completely irrelevant to your progress. Whatever metrics you pick to monitor you must do it daily so that you build up an average of your progress, which is a much better measure to gauge results.

Once you have a few weeks of data to review you will get a really clear picture of how things are progressing, or not. This means you can make effective adjustments, be it reducing calories, adding in an extra gym session or increasing your steps. Here's a very important point to note though; in 90% of client cases that I work with, it's hardly ever the calorie intake that is the issue if they are sticking to the plan. Most of the time we will see that the activity has dropped off as a result of the diet and so we need to go back to the 'I' step to improve.

The important thing is that whatever you find needs improving you go back and make an adjustment and then monitor it. Eventually, you'll find a sweet spot where you continue to make progress, and then you keep things the same until you see a plateau. Remember that just because you are making improvements, it doesn't mean that you can stop monitoring your data. Inevitably you'll see a slowdown and you'll need to know why this has happened.

57. GET TO THE CHOPPER! – PROCESS IS NOTHING WITHOUT SUPPORT SYSTEMS

The C.A.L.O.R.I.E. system is an incredibly effective process for creating and managing your fat-loss journey. However, the process is useless without the systems to support it.

Don't believe me? Then think back to every single diet that you've done and failed at. They all had really fancy and shiny processes to help you lose body fat but how many helped you develop a support system that taught you how to implement the process and cope with any errors and issues that came up?

I'm willing to bet absolutely zero, or you wouldn't be reading this.

Most diet programmes will give you a plan, then just expect you to follow it perfectly. That's only the beginning though. Any fool with a calculator and a food database can write a diet for someone as it's basically a calorie balancing equation. Even these people understand the importance of a calorie deficit.

The real skill comes in equipping yourself with all the tools for the job. My favourite film ever is *Commando* with Arnold Schwarzenegger. The memorable scene on the beach, where he suits up from his swimming trunks into a battle-ready killing machine loaded with guns, is how I want you to prepare for your mission to lose body fat.

If you haven't seen the film, google 'Commando beach gear-up scene' and you'll get the idea.

Of course, Arnold's character may have been able to rescue his daughter and kill a lot of baddies with only half the guns, but it would have been much tougher. If he'd rocked up in just his trunks and a motivation to succeed, then I'm pretty sure that he wouldn't have even got past the first guard post and may instead be running for a chopper to airlift him out, like in the movie, *Predator*.

This is the issue with diets in general. We all rock up on the beach at the start with all the motivation in the world but then barely get past the first guard post because that's the first real challenge. Most people give up on their diet when they face a serious challenge that puts them out of their comfort zone and messes up their routine. Some make it through but then get splatted by the guy with the machine gun at the next gate, because their initial motivation has been severely cut down by the first challenge.

I'm going to equip you with all the equipment you need to splat all the bad guys – those things that pop up to try to stop you succeeding. The weapons of choice are habit and adaptation techniques that I've used with clients over the last ten years and have been extremely successful. You may not need all of them but you'll have them just in case, because you never know when the *boss* baddie will emerge.

58. BANKING AND SPENDING

The first four steps of the C.A.L.O.R.I.E. system are creating your meals. At the very basic level this gives you a day planner to eat the same amount and size of meals every day.

A great many diets do this and give you set meals; however, I have found that 99% of my clients do not live like this, eating the same amount of meals, and size of meals, every day of the week. The majority of people eat a different amount at the weekend as they work in the week and have weekends off with their family. Others who work at weekends have days off in the week and eat more or less the same on those days.

It's never helpful to try to force people to eat more meals than they want, or conversely to eat much less than they normally do, but this is how many diets are constructed. They just don't get that you may want a varying meal schedule on some days of the week.

This is where banking and spending come in. Earlier in the book I discussed that it was the average calories over the week that matter and not so much the daily calories. We want to be in a deficit on average over seven to twenty-eight days and having one day of surplus calories won't matter if you're in a deficit for the rest of the week.

Banking calories is where you anticipate that you will eat more on a weekend or other day, which may be a birthday party or a special event. With the best willpower in the world we all know that if we go to these events our Muncher brain is going to give us cues to eat the cake or the buffet, because that's the social environment we are in. We want to relax at such events and trying to stick to a diet is a stress trigger that brings out the Muncher with desires to eat nice food to make us feel better.

With this truth accepted we can plan for it. Here is an example of a banking strategy for our 100 kg man who knows that 2,400 calories per day is a deficit amount for him from the first step in the C.A.L.O.R.I.E. system.

	Normal cals eaten	Banking cals eaten	Accumulated balance
Mon	2,400	2,000	+400
Tues	2,400	2,000	+800
Wed	2,400	2,000	+1,200
Thurs	2,400	2,000	+1,600
Fri	2,400	2,000	+2,000
Sat	2,400	3,400	+1,000
Sun	2,400	3,400	0
Total	16,800	16,800	

You'll see that through the week in the normal pattern he eats the same each day, however, there's no consideration for the weekend. This leaves him open to a risk of overeating if there's a special event as there's nothing held in reserve.

In the second example he restricts his food slightly, maybe by reducing his snacks or meals in the day, through the week in order to bank up a significant number of calories for the weekend. This means he can eat more with his family during a weekend break.

The total calories consumed in the week are exactly the same, he just creates more of a deficit in the beginning of the week and overeats at the end of the week.

Due to this he may see a slight body weight increase at the end of the week due to the volume of food he has eaten, however, this will be offset by the deficit at the beginning of the week. Overall, he will see a drop in bodyweight on average over the month by sticking to this plan each week.

Banking and spending is a key skill to master if you want to allow yourself more flexibility on your diet and in your life. Building up the buffer with the extra restriction allows you a reserve amount that you can dip into at any time, if you have a need for it, with the confidence that you are still on target for the week.

You may see this method referred to as calorie cycling, or the 5:2 diet. Where banking and spending differs is that you can log your banking over a 4-week period in order to save up a very big surplus for a holiday whereas calorie cycling, or 5:2, are firmly fixed on a week view in general.

I've used banking with clients to prepare for a big holiday where they know they will be eating more for a week or two. We plan out a three-week higher deficit so that when they go away, they are confident of the buffer. They may gain a little bit of weight back but crucially they never go above their starting weight. This point is important to note because many people go on holiday after a crash diet and when they return, they have gained loads of weight. Even worse, they continue the overeating into their time back, which further ruins their weight-loss efforts. If you have fully prepared beforehand then the fallout from a week or two off is minimal and this gives you a positive boost on your return.

59. PLANNING TO FAIL

This may seem weird, as all the way through the book I've been telling you that if you follow the plan you'll never fail and never need another diet plan, because you'll be prepared and have all the weapons at your disposal.

Well, 99% of the time this is true and being prepared is essential for success, but you also need to be prepared for that 1% of times where things conspire against you to play cruel tricks on your mind and time management, so that you find the idea of diving into a tray of cakes very appealing.

Planning to fail incorporates two elements.

1. **Planned failure**
   This is similar to banking and spending, however, you incorporate into your normal daily calories a cheat, or junk-type, meal. For example, our 100 kg man may have 800 calories left in his day of 2,000 and instead of having his 2 meals of 400 calories, he opts instead for a pizza or a

takeaway. This is food that he hadn't planned on eating but incorporates into his normal calorie intake because he feels like having them after a stressful day, or because he just fancies a pizza.

2. **Life conspiracy**
   We've all had the experience of what seems like life conspiring against us. No matter what we do in a day to try to stick to our routine, it just doesn't happen the way we planned it and for whatever reason we can't eat the foods we had planned out. Whether it results in a small binge or just overeating because the food that's available is higher calorie, it's important not to get upset about this.

Many people will mistakenly believe that by overeating in a day or weekend they have destroyed their diet progress, and this is 'proven' to them by a slight weight gain the next day. It's important to recognise that the weight gain is absolutely not fat being stored as this just does not happen so quickly, and certainly not from just a few thousand calories surplus. It takes over 7,000 surplus calories to store 1 kg of fat and unless you've really gone to town on the food it's unlikely you've eaten this much.

Even then it's much more likely that a huge volume of overeaten food will be excreted in the main rather than stored totally as fat from a day's overeating. It takes a sustained eating habit to start to store significant fat, and so if you have just had one or two days where you've gone off the rails it's important to get back onto your plan as soon as possible to return the body to a deficit, and you will find that the weight drops again in the next few days.

Planning to fail means that you accept that sometimes your Muncher brain will pop up and score a win when you are least expecting it. It's really important that you don't get angry at yourself or the situation as this creates a stress response and this only causes the Muncher to resurface to try to make you feel better by suggesting more overeating of your favourite treats.

Instead, accept that it has happened, understand that life sometimes doesn't go to plan and then move on, maybe making a note of why the trigger situation happened and how you could avoid it next time.

This brings us nicely on to the next skill.

60. WORKING WITH YOUR BRAINS

That isn't a typo. You may recall back in Section 1 I introduced you to the idea of the three brains that everyone has: The Muncher, Tivor and the Robot. Muncher always pops up when you are stressed or tired and most of the time suggests eating foods that you would prefer not to eat when you are fully calm and rested. Hunger will also trigger the Muncher to come out as its purpose is to protect you from threat, and hunger eventually becomes a threat to your bodily functions.

It's impossible to fight the Muncher for an extended period. It is a much more powerful creature than Tivor, who is your logical, rational brain. With each resistance you put up the Muncher absorbs it and becomes stronger, eventually overpowering you, and the strength it has accumulated explodes onto your plate in a massive binge.

Fighting is not on the menu and so our best bet is to work with it and keep it docile and obedient. This is why we build in elements, such as the banking and spending technique, as you can have an inner monologue between your brains promising the Muncher a big feed if he goes to sleep until the higher calorie day.

Many diets will tell you that certain foods are forbidden, or that they are bad, or carry an increased sinful value compared to others. This does not help the brains work together because essentially your logical Tivor brain has put the Muncher in a prison, which it will eventually break out of.

By eliminating some of your favourite foods the diet plan has removed the element of choice from you, which works against your brain. Although some people do have the willpower to completely take out nice treats from their diet for an extended period and eat completely 'clean', these are the minority and are generally those who end up in massive rebounds.

Everyone breaks, remember that.

61. IDENTIFY YOURSELF – LIVE THE LIFE OF THE PERSON YOU WANT TO BE

In order to work with your brains, you need to think about changing your identity. This isn't a new passport and a trip to Venezuela but casting votes for your leaner lifestyle. Many people I meet on a weight-loss journey will say that they are trying to lose a certain number of kilograms. This means that they still identify themselves as the heavier person they are trying to change. In order to facilitate long-term change we need to think like the person we want to become.

I used to smoke when I was a teenager. I tried to quit unsuccessfully a number of times until I realised where I was going wrong. I never had any cigarettes on me and I always told people I was trying to quit.

This may sound stupid but hear me out. It was only when I started carrying cigarettes with me all the time, and telling people that I was a non-smoker, that I actually managed to quit. Why was this?

Simply, I gave myself the choice. I could light up a cigarette anytime I liked. I had them to hand at all times, which meant that I hadn't restricted my access to them. I made consistent choices and cast votes for being a non-smoker rather than someone who was trying to quit.

Key Point

If you always tell people that you are on a diet, or that you're trying to lose weight, then you're identifying as someone who overeats. Which is why you've gained weight. This is a lead into the prison and ultimately leads to a break on the diet as you will always identify as that overweight person who overeats, which means that being overweight is the normal state and losing weight is the unusual state.

If instead, you decide on living a leaner lifestyle and follow a diet within a deficit in order to live this life, you are no longer someone who overeats. You are simply someone eating a certain number of calories a day to maintain and develop a leaner body.

You need to cast votes every day for your new leaner lifestyle. Every situation you encounter you need to be thinking, "what does the leaner me choose to do?" Note I use '*does*' not '*would*'. Would implies that you are still in your old state and not your new leaner lifestyle state.

For example,

- Do you take the lift or the stairs?
- Do you have a lazy ten minutes sitting on the sofa surfing Facebook or do you take your phone and walk around the block surfing Facebook?

- Do you park your car right outside the supermarket, or do you park across the car park so you can get some extra steps in?

All these don't really impact your normal lifestyle that much, but they are very small adjustments that are votes for a leaner person's behaviour. Eventually, by always choosing the leaner lifestyle option this identity becomes your standard identity and you remove your identity as an overeating, underactive, overweight person. I don't mean any insult by that, but the reason you've gained weight *is* a lack of activity combined with more food than you need.

The more votes that you cast for your desired lifestyle the easier it will become to work with your brains, by resetting their perception of what they see as the normal you. This makes it easier for you to dismiss actions that take you back to your old life, as these will now be unusual actions rather than normal activity.

Activity – casting votes

Get a piece of paper and draw a line down the middle. On the left at the top write 'Votes for a leaner lifestyle' and on the right 'Votes for my old lifestyle'. You can also download a template from www.bkmnutrition.com/ivotelean

Over the course of a week I want you to log all the votes you have made for the two lifestyles.

Every time you vote for your old life look at the vote and ask yourself why this wasn't a vote for the leaner lifestyle and how it could be tweaked for your leaner lifestyle.

Bear in mind I am not looking for total lifestyle change here, votes for your leaner life may include

- I had two beers instead of three tonight
- I only had half a portion of chips
- I swapped my crisps for Snack a Jacks

They are little wins that set you on the path, though of course I also would like to see you walking up the stairs and making healthier food choices. If you need a hand with adjusting any of your votes to leaner ones then post in the Target Lean Lifestyle group on Facebook and I'll help with the solution. If you've had some wins that you want to share, then also let me know. I genuinely do like seeing people get some positive results.

62. THE LANGUAGE OF DIETING – TALKING YOURSELF INTO ACTION

I often meet people who tell me that they should go on a diet and they don't know why they have gained weight. More often than not this is a closed conversation. They don't actually have the desire to go on a diet and they probably do know deep down why they have gained weight.

The language that they use is one of defeat and is negatively charged, there's no solution just a problem. This is quite common and it's not that the person is an inherently negative person, they just are unable to formulate a way out. This does stem from the three pressure points, namely confusion and frustration, but also their perception that all diets need to be prisons.

You may have done this yourself.

"I should go to the gym or exercise more."

"I should lose some weight."

"I should eat healthier."

All these are negative leads of a desired behaviour followed by a reason or an excuse as to why the action doesn't happen.

"I should go to the gym more, but I never have time due to my job."

"I should lose some weight, but I don't know what to eat."

"I should eat healthier, but it's so expensive to eat right."

Despite the fact that they have even stated the reason why they aren't performing the action in their reason, there's no effort made to change it. It's an excuse for their actions not a reason.

Using certain words can bring a negative and failure mentality to your dieting efforts. I want you to start rethinking your language that you use as this will actually set you up for action to change.

Language is also is relevant to our vote-casting for our lives and is definitely something that defines us in our new identity.

For example:

Undesirable Identity Language.	Desirable Identity Language.
I should go to the gym more, but I never have time and can't be bothered.	I could go to the gym more if I went with a friend to keep me accountable or I enlisted a personal trainer.
I should eat healthier, but it's so expensive and I have no idea how to cook.	I could eat healthier if instead of a takeaway I bought my Saturday night meal from an online food prep company that delivers all the ingredients and instructions to my door.
I don't know why I keep gaining weight as I hardly eat anything.	I could find out how I keep gaining weight by tracking my food intake every day.
I should be more active, but my job is desk based and I'm sitting down all day.	I could be more active at work; if I took the stairs instead of the lift and set my alarm every hour for a three-minute walk around the office.
I can't lose weight I have no idea where to start.	I could lose weight if I enlisted a nutritionist to help me plan out my food and lifestyle.

Generally, if you find yourself justifying an undesirable action with a reason then this can be adjusted by changing your habits using the vote sheet, and the language you use can help you find the solution.

Key point

Positive language will always include an action and negative language always includes inaction or a weakness.

This does sound like a lot of psychobabble and I'll understand if at first you dismiss it as a stupid idea but it's a very powerful tool when done right. We are generally averse to changing our behaviour and new things tend to bring out a defensive response, which is why the negative language is used in the first place. It's a defence of our current position.

A lot of people won't even vocalise a reason as to why they can't do their 'should' action, they'll just state it and that's what they perceive as their accepted state and are resigned to staying there.

Positive actions come from a positive mindset and your mindset is established from the language that you use in your internal conversations and with others. It's a Robot function to either immediately think *should* or *could* and therefore to make this always a *could* option there needs to be repeated conscious thought towards the *could*.

The more that you think about this action the more you will see other people performing the *should* action in their conversations with you. Now that you are aware of it hopefully you will start to make small changes in your own lifestyle. Remember that the *could* options don't need to be world changing. Set a realistic alternate option and grow it from there. "I should exercise more" becomes "I could exercise more by walking up one flight of stairs before taking the lift" then becomes two flights, then three. The more votes that you cast the easier it is to cast bigger votes for that life.

Activity – changing the language

This is an ongoing challenge for you. Whenever you find yourself saying 'I should do ...'

Stop and think about saying instead 'I could do ... if I ...'

I've found that when challenging clients to do this they've figured out the solution to a lot of their issues with their lifestyle changes themselves. You may find that you need help from a nutritionist or personal trainer for some weight-loss solutions but finding that solution is the first step.

Download a template for changing your language from www.bkmnutrition.com/language to get you started. If you need a hand figuring out the solution, then feel free to ask for some help in my Target Lean Lifestyle group on Facebook.

63. HAVE A VERY VOCAL WORD WITH YOURSELF

You'll have to be careful with this technique, as if you do it too much in public it's likely you'll be taken away by the people in white coats. Internal monologues are OK in theory, but they are only thoughts. Thoughts are useless unless they become actions and we need to talk ourselves into action.

A self-checking chat can be a very useful tool to reset the Muncher's desire for snacking and nice treats and also set the boundaries for the day.

The Muncher is a great deal stronger than your logical Tivor brain and so if he wakes up in a hungry state it can be difficult to manage those thoughts as well as the other 1,000 things that you may think about in the next 10 minutes. This then allows the Muncher to sneak in the back and before you know it, you're snacking on biscuits while organising your diary.

Vocal self-checks are an important check in many industries for avoiding accidents; they reinforce the command or decision and confirm it's the course of action. If you've ever seen any US submarine film, then you'll see this in action with the commands dictated by the captain being repeated by the helmsman before diving a certain depth or turning a certain way. You may also do this already and not know it. Have you ever stood by your door and performed a vocal self-check of "I've got my keys, my phone, my wallet"?

How we apply this to working with your Muncher brain is as follows: if you suddenly get an inkling for something snack orientated, then you can have a quick conversation with yourself.

"A doughnut would be nice, but let's wait until I've finished my housework and then I can enjoy it with a cup of tea."

"I think it would be better to have that pack of crisps with my lunch so I'm full up afterwards, rather than right now."

The conversation isn't a denial of the snack but a postponement, which is a bargain with the Muncher to wait a while before you have the snack. In most cases, unless you are ravenously hungry, this will be an acceptable compromise.

It's important that you don't try to use this method to attempt to trick the Muncher in an effort to forget the craving, as it will immediately see through this trick and come back more insistent. It is you, remember, it will know when you are lying. That doesn't mean you can't postpone again later if you both want to. Resistance is never a good option, but negotiation and compromise work well.

64. RIDING THE WAVE – CONTROLLING EATING CRAVINGS WITH LOGICAL THOUGHT

I've never been much good at surfing. Being a short, thick-set bodybuilder, my balance is not great, especially on a two-metre plank in the sea. However, the principles of surfing can be used quite nicely in this technique.

I referred to the neurotransmitter, dopamine, in Section 1. You may recall that it's the driving force behind most of our actions that we believe will yield a positive or rewarding result. However, positive and rewarding don't always go together. For example, dopamine drives the gambling urge in anticipation of a rewarding event in a win, but more often than not the gambling results in a less-than-positive outcome.

The same is true when we look at our drive for eating. If I asked you to think about your favourite chocolate bar for ten seconds, you'd probably get a small motivational drive to eat it because your previous experience of eating that bar produced a rewarding feeling.

Now think about the food you really don't like much; mine is sprouts. When I think about sprouts, I really don't get a drive to eat them. They are not rewarding to me and this is why I have zero motivation to eat them. I do sometimes eat them if they are included in a roast dinner though as I am a nutritionist and I understand the benefit of eating green vegetables. Combined with a roast dinner and some gravy they are OK to eat, just.

We can override our negative thoughts about a food or action by justifying it in another way, usually a logical thought. There is no real dopamine release in response to seeing the food, so we have to motivate ourselves consciously.

In comparison, when we see a food that we really like we have no trouble getting a nice fat dopamine spike, and this can often be strong enough to override logical thought and drive us to commit unspeakable acts of gluttony while our logical brain looks on, powerless to resist.

Dopamine drives the Muncher and gives it strength. If we are unprepared for it then we have no defence. This is where 'riding the wave' comes in.

As soon as we see a food that we like we will get a hit of dopamine to eat it. If we are full and have just eaten it's unlikely that we will act on it because our satiety hormones have kicked in to tell us that we are full and so our hunger response is minimal. We have more logical strength and from an instinctual aspect we have no reason to eat more, as we have just eaten and are full.

However, when we are trying to lose weight, we are rarely in a state of complete fullness apart from maybe in the ten minutes immediately after a meal, which means that our hunger will be fuelled by the release of dopamine and spike with it, creating a huge desire to eat the food in front of us. If that food has a high perceived value in terms of both calorie content and pleasure, then it's incredibly hard to resist.

We still possess logical thought for a time until the Muncher wears us down, so we get on our mental surfboard and ride the dopamine wave while it peaks and at the same time remove the stimulus – the food – from our vision. You will never be able to resist if you sit looking at a plate of doughnuts for long, but if you take them away then the stimulus will start to subside and the wave of dopamine will diminish after five to ten minutes.

If you've successfully ridden the wave then your desire to eat that food will disappear, however, you may still have a smaller general hunger sensation and so it might be prudent to have one of your low-impact snacks from your LEAN Matrix to hand, just in case.

Riding the wave works well for unexpected, random stimuli that pop up in the day. It won't be effective against real hunger drivers, which are caused by low calorie availability or low blood sugar, and so it's important to assess whether your hunger drive was only brought on by the sight of the food or you were hungry already and the sight of the food enhanced it.

You can see a video about riding the wave at
www.bkmnutrition.com/ridingthewave

65. A MESSAGE IN A BOTTLE – LESSONS FROM YOUR PAST LIFE

No one knows you like yourself. You may have been told to forget the past as it's in the past, however, as far as making progress with your fat loss goes, we absolutely want to remember our past actions.

One of the first tasks that we ask Target Lean members to do is to write a letter to themselves. In this they detail why they think that their diets didn't work for them in the past as well as which parts worked for them. Although the reasons will lead back to the three pressure points, we need to identify the specific reasons for them so that we can change them. Whether it be further education on nutrition, proper routines and habit coaching, or just new ideas for boring meals, something let them down and until they themselves are honest about those reasons they will never accept the solutions, or the methods, that the programme teaches.

It's important for the member to have the desire for change in order for them to accept the knowledge and techniques to enable that change. Many weight-loss programmes are directional and dictatorial in their approach in that they have a rigid system that their members must follow. For long-lasting change to occur the plan must have flexibility and be adaptable to the person's changing circumstances. Assuming that the reason the person failed to lose weight in the past was that they just ate too much is too simplistic a view.

Of course, the person ate more than they expended, but why did that happen? Was it that they didn't know how to work out calories? Maybe they were using their food app incorrectly. Perhaps they had all their meals out ready and they just weren't able to eat them due to work or family commitments, which led to having to eat other food on the go.

Writing the letter will identify this and it's a very important and useful step that I recommend you do every few months while you are trying to improve your body shape. It will reaffirm how you are progressing and identify key barriers that still stand in your way.

Activity – write yourself a letter

This doesn't need to be an epic piece of literature. A guide to writing it is as follows:

*Dear ****,*

When I tried to lose weight for (insert goal or reason and the date) there were a few issues that got in the way such as (reasons why you couldn't stick to the diet). I think these were due to (issues you think influenced your difficulties).

I think I COULD change (first reason) by (help you think you need or thing you think that you need to do).

Repeat for all reasons

That's it. Then stick it on your fridge as a reminder of the things that got in your way before. The more conscious you are of your past problems the less likely you'll make them by mistake again, and it's more likely that you can use it on your vote sheet to help change your habits.

This is a *could* letter. Rather than wallowing in your own self-pity about your failure, document the issues and make a plan for action.

Not sure what things you may need to change? Post in the Target Lean Lifestyle group on Facebook. I'll give you a few pointers.

66. IF THIS ... THEN – CREATING A PLAN TO GET YOU BACK TO THE FUTURE

"Marty, you aren't thinking 4th Dimensionally."

Doc. Emmett Brown

('Back to the Future')

We often think of diet progress in a linear fashion. We start a diet, we do some exercise stuff, eat some lower-calorie stuff and at the end we come out leaner.

Good in theory, and the people who bang on about, "it's all down to calorie deficit," love that kind of straight-line thinking. While losing weight is about maintaining a calorie deficit, it's never that simple.

Like I said in Section 1, if a business coach told you the way to make more money is to, "sell more stuff and spend less money," then you'd fire him immediately. Why, though – that's what you need to do in order to make more money, surely?

There's obviously much more to it than that. Having a Plan B in business is absolutely essential. Ten years of owning my own gym has taught me that very rarely do things go to plan however meticulously you plan them.

In order to successfully create and maintain a calorie deficit you need to have fall-back options planned.

When Marty messed up his timeline in *Back to the Future*, he had a DeLorean to travel back in time to put it right. Unfortunately, we don't have that luxury and so we need to think a little fourth dimensionally to anticipate future events and make a correction in our timeline to get back to the right future, and not one where we have demolished a million calories of carbs and ice cream.

If this ...then, planning can start with the letter that you write to yourself. You will have created a list of past issues that you experienced and so we can easily start to plan out a solution using those events as a base model.

For example, one issue I had was that I would sit down on my sofa with a tub of Pringles and pile through them one by one until I reached the end and had consumed over 500 calories.

Therefore, my 'If this ... then' protocol reads like this:

"*If* I find myself wanting to snack on Pringles, *then* I will pour some into a bowl and take the bowl out to the sofa and leave the Pringles in the cupboard so that I have a natural break cue to stop me."

By using the break cues technique, I was successfully able to prevent myself overeating on snack foods. Break cues is covered in the next habit.

Another one that came up regularly was that I would very often get home late from work and be very tired and not want to make myself a meal. This would lead to me ordering an Uber Eats.

Therefore, I installed an 'If this ... then' to deal with it.

"*If* I come home late and am too tired to eat, which makes me think about a takeaway, *then* I will instead eat one of the microwave meal pots that I have in the freezer."

Both these came from the letter that I wrote to myself. I used the vote sheet to track my successes and failures, and over time I increased my number of successes. Now these are routine habits for me. If I want a takeaway, it's a conscious choice I make and not a fall-back option. If I want to eat more Pringles I can, but it's my choice to do so and not my instinctual or subconscious snacking drive.

Key Point

Choice is a key element in a successful long-term identity change. Choosing to indulge yourself in a few treats now and again is normal and healthy behaviour.

67. HABITS – CREATING AND ELIMINATING FRICTION

There are many habits that you can use to help you lose weight and live a leaner lifestyle. While a lot of these will depend on your individual circumstances, there are a few common ones that I've come across repeatedly that are easy to implement and are applicable to most people in some way.

The key thing to remember when trying to build a good habit is to create more friction for bad habits and reduce friction for good habits. We follow a path of least resistance, and so if a good or desirable habit requires a lot of steps or hoops to jump through, we are more likely to divert to the undesirable habits. These are generally very low on friction or we would not do them repeatedly. Conversely good or desirable habits normally have some degree of 'doing something else', which makes them more time-consuming or more difficult, which is why we don't do them often.

For example:

- Having a bowl of chocolate treats on the living room table or in plain sight in the kitchen or workplace means that it's very easy to snack on chocolate. Swap the chocolate for fruit and it becomes easier to snack on fruit
- Having pre-prepared healthy, low-calorie meals in the fridge that you can eat cold, or microwave in four minutes, means that it's easier and quicker to heat up a low-calorie meal than order a takeaway if you can't be bothered to cook

Key point

The more opportunities that you allow to be present that can break your diet the more chance that you will break eventually. Remember, your Muncher brain is instinctual and can override your logical Tivor brain if given the chance to. We want zero friction for desirable habits and huge friction for undesirable habits.

The great thing about reducing friction is that eventually these desirable habits become installed in your Robot brain and become instinctual, so you automatically default to these as the normal behaviour because they require less thinking and are very easy to do.

Here are a few examples of habits that can help you reduce or add friction where needed and can be added to your daily routine very easily.

68. BREAK CUES

One of the biggest black holes for overeating is the time when you're sitting on the sofa in the evening, with a feast of snacks in front of you, and you munch through them while watching endless TV.

My undoing in this regard is Pringles. If I sit with the whole tube I just eat until the whole tube is gone. That's 1,000 calories!

You will have your own black hole snack, and this might be something from the no man's land in your LEAN Matrix, or even a low-calorie snack that you massively overeat on from the low-impact snacks box. Whatever it is, you need to rein that in, and break cues provide that essential tool.

Instead of sitting down with the whole tube of Pringles, or a big box of Quality Street, tip some into a bowl in the kitchen, then put the tube or box out of sight right at the top of the cupboard or somewhere equally annoying to get to. Then sit down, watch the TV and snack through the bowl. Of course, the bowl shouldn't be a three-litre type; a small cereal bowl should be the limit. If it's chocolate, then even smaller is better as eight cubes of a caramel big bar is about 300 calories, and they will be gone in no time.

You'll reach the end of the bowl after a while and then you have to make a conscious decision to get up, go to the kitchen and navigate the top of the cupboard to pour out more snacks and go back to your seat.

All this is friction, and if you're relaxing it's quite likely you can't be bothered to get up. You most likely won't be hungry and so the only driver is a hedonic desire to eat, which is most likely suppressed. You'll have had your dopamine reward spike and with that and hunger satisfied and friction to getting more food, it's likely you'll just settle down.

Think about the opposite situation like Christmas where it's common for families to drape their living rooms with chocolate and have big boxes of treats within easy reach. No wonder January diet programmes do so well – they are primed to feed off your guilt for the gold medal in uncontrolled eating you've just won over Christmas.

Without a conscious break cue for your eating you will overeat. Now I know what you may be thinking: "Not me, I have control and I will stop when I feel like it." When snacking has been studied using Pringles as the food, researchers placed a red Pringle at different points down the tube. You'd think that people would just eat regardless and stop when they're full, however, when people reached the red Pringle they stopped shortly after, regardless of where the red Pringle was placed. What this means is that when our brain receives an unusual cue that breaks our momentum, we tend to re-evaluate the situation.

I'm not expecting you to place a red Pringle in your snacks, although this may help now you've read this. However, if we place a natural 'stop' signal in our snacks, then we will break our subconscious eating patterns just for a moment and you can actually assess if you are still hungry or not.

You can see a video on break cues on my website at www.bkmnutrition.com/breakcues

69. ANCHORING

Anchoring is when you immediately associate a cue with an action. For example, the smell of fresh bread from a bakery may trigger a memory of baked goods and how nice they are, and all of a sudden you're in the shop buying doughnuts wondering what the hell just happened.

Anchors can be positive and negative and it's something used extensively in hypnotherapy and Neuro Linguistic Programming techniques to create a feeling or emotion that leads to an action. How anchoring affects you in terms of your eating habits is as follows.

You come home from work, you put your bag down and go into the kitchen and immediately go to the cupboard to get a snack. This tends to be a chocolate or other quick hit of calories. This is your daily routine, but it only happens on workdays because the anchor is created from the accumulation of all your activities leading up to that point.

When I've worked with clients on their daily routines I can see these anchors straight away. They want to stop snacking on chocolate but can't seem to resist it when they get home from work.

The anchor build-up may look like this:

Get home from work (cue) ➽ put bag down (cue 2) ➽ go into kitchen (cue 3) ➽ think about a snack (thought) ➽ eat chocolate (action).

The stacking up of the cues in this situation means that the end result of eating chocolate is the habitual outcome of all the actions or cues before it. The anchor created is that coming home from work is associated with eating chocolate.

However, when the same person comes home from a day out on a weekend, the cues could be different and lead to a different end action. It's important to identify all the steps of this routine, which may be subconscious, so you can assess where you can install a break in the routine and establish a new anchor.

For example, in the series of events above there are a number of build-up triggers:

1. Get home from work
2. Put bag down
3. Go into kitchen

It's impossible to change the 'get home from work' as you always have to come home, but the next two can be tweaked. I have had a number of clients that followed this type of routine to various degrees and we tweaked it as follows:

1. Get home from work
2. Go into bedroom
3. Put bag down in bedroom
4. Change into comfies
5. Collect washing from bedroom
6. Go into kitchen and put washing on
7. Think about a snack while putting washing on

The break in the routine installs a number of extra steps into the routine to create friction to the snacking on chocolate end result. It also installs a good habit in that they perform a routine action that helps with the house maintenance. Over all this time they have time to think about their snack and we made sure that they had low-calorie snacks such as fruit or Snack a Jacks within easy reach once they'd put the washing on.

This is a routine that creates a new anchor for the coming home routine. What about if the person is *really* hungry though when they get home? Well then, we had another anchor for that, and it involved always having a ready meal in the fridge ready to cook within three minutes and it went like this:

1. Get home
2. ***Don't*** put bag down
3. Go into kitchen
4. Get ready meal out of the fridge
5. Put bag down (optional)
6. Put ready meal into microwave

7. Go upstairs, put bag into bedroom and change into comfies while meal is cooking
8. Come downstairs to eat ready meal

There's also an alternative option for this involving a cold meal, like a sandwich or salad, in the fridge, in which case the anchor would be:

1. Get home from work
2. Put bag in bedroom
3. Change into comfies
4. Bring washing down
5. Put washing in machine
6. Get cold meal out of fridge and eat

You may notice some common threads here.

- We removed the trigger anchor of putting the bag down immediately when they came home, which was then the signal to progress to the next stage of the routine
- Instead, the bag was put into the bedroom, which was a change of location for the next stage of the routine
- We changed the client into comfies in *all* of the situations, which removed the state of the person from being in work mode, and into a new state of being relaxed at home
- We reduced friction for the easier option; the ready meal was in the fridge and needed

only three minutes to cook while the person did something else to occupy their mind Alternatively, they could opt for the cold meal already in the fridge

In all of the cases we broke the original routine and location, and state anchors of the person, so that there was no subconscious reference for the next event. Over time, the changing of state into comfies became the signal to eat healthier foods containing fewer calories overall.

Work with your brain, look at the undesirable actions that you perform and what are the sequence of events leading up to the action. You'll find that some people will say to overweight people, "why don't you just stop eating chocolate when you come home?" It's of course very easy in theory, but when we have habits and routines installed in our brain we have to address those to change the outcome.

Everything is involved in the process. Music can be a powerful anchor for setting a mind state; boxers and MMA fighters don't walk out to lullabies, and babies don't fall asleep listening to heavy metal. If the music in your car is setting you up for the undesirable action, then change what you listen to when you're driving home or to work.

Similarly, a change of clothes can be a powerful anchor; you don't go to work in your pyjamas, and you don't relax in your business suit. Changing your state of dress changes your mindset for the next actions.

Activity

Terminator Timeline – identify your undesirable actions and work back to find your cues

On a piece of paper in landscape, write on the left-hand side, a list of all your undesirable habits or actions that you do.

Then working across the page list every action or cue that precedes the previous one. Eventually you will arrive at the origin cue. Once you have that all mapped out, look at the things you can actually change in the sequence. It's likely that most of the time the origin cue will be unchangeable such as 'coming home from work' so you'll need to look at the next ones along the list. Think about things you can change.

1. The location where you do things
2. The clothes that you are wearing
3. The people that you are with
4. The music that you are listening to

Once you've got all the stages mapped out then create a Terminator Timeline branching off from the original so that you can change the future. Hopefully, this doesn't involve murdering people with an Uzi, but you gotta do what you gotta do.

(Jokes, "don't murder people please, it might be bad for book sales.")

Remember that the alternate timelines need to be easier to do and involve changes of states where possible and can't include elements from the previous timeline if possible. We want to change the outcome of the future by adjusting the events leading up to it.

Create friction for the undesirable habits and reduce friction for the desirable habits. Where possible stack up new desirable habits like I did in the example of changing into comfies and putting the washing on. These are positive habits for both relaxation and getting mundane jobs done in the house. Double Win!

70. SELF-SABOTAGE

By now you have a number of very powerful tools to help you with your diet; you know how to calculate your calories, allocate them to your day, incorporate foods that you like into your diet and how to cope with situations that come up that may force you off plan.

Let's now deal with you. You can be your own worst enemy when trying to lose weight, and I'm talking about self-sabotage.

There are five important areas that you need to consider.

1. Removing negative cues from your life
2. Not revisiting places of previous bad experience
3. Ensuring adequate sleep and rest times
4. Setting unrealistic time constraints
5. Thinking about the goal and not the process

Some of these I've covered in part previously in the book so let's have a recap.

1. Removing negative cues from your life

Leaving temptation in sight is an often overlooked and easy to fix negative cue. In studies done on office workers, the ones who had sweets placed on their desk, in direct sight, ate much more than those where the sweets were in the drawer and even more compared to when the sweets were placed across the office involving a walk to get them. Remember to increase friction for your snacking black holes.

One thing I see repeatedly come up is the 'drive through cue'. This involves the person's daily route taking them past McDonald's or similar drive through where it's incredibly easy to pull in to get a hot chocolate or calorie-laden coffee. Taking a slightly different route to work or home can reduce these cues massively. Think riding the wave if you can't change your route, or already have a lower-calorie drink in your car to reduce friction for the lower-calorie option.

2. Negative location anchors

If you are a recovering alcoholic you don't go into pubs, if you are a reformed gambler you avoid casinos. Many people walk into a fast food joint with the intention of buying a salad, but because their previous anchors are for a burger and chips, that's what they come out with. Avoid negative location anchors completely. Even if you haven't been there for ages the anchor will still exist to a degree and you may find it resurfaces with a vengeance very quickly. If your previous life involved bingeing on certain foods at certain restaurants, then it's best to avoid them until you have firmly established your new leaner identity.

3. Adequate sleep and rest times

There is a belief that poor sleep can cause fat gain. This is not true in its entirety as lack of sleep does not then mean you gain body fat. However, poor sleep does mean that your logical functions are impaired and as a result of this you can make poor food choices. You'll generally go for easier to prepare food because you want the path of least resistance, which normally manifests in takeaways or fast food. Ensuring that you are getting at least six hours sleep a day will help this. I know that many people recommend eight hours or more; while this may be optimal it is not always possible. I have a young son, at the time of writing he is three years old. Six hours sleep to me is like a unicorn. To help remedy this I have thirty-minute power naps during the day. Although this is not going to replace deep REM sleep, it does go some way to offering protection against more impulsive behaviour.

4. Time constraining your goals without good reason

A classic behaviour study on time constrained goals vs open goals involved the classic candle and tacks problem. The problem was that the students were presented with:

- A candle
- A box of tacks
- A cork board

The task at hand was to secure the candle to the board with a secondary goal of ensuring no wax dripped onto the floor. One group was given a ten-minute window, and the other an open goal just to complete the task.

The time constraint forced the first group to think about the goal. Fixing the candle to the cork board became the number one priority. They tried fixing the candle to the board, resting the candle on the tacks and all sorts of other solutions before finally stumbling on the actual solution that solved both the issues.

An interesting result was that the non-time-constrained group came across the solution much faster, possibly due to the lack of a time limit, and they had time to consider the process rather than the goal.

The solution?

Empty the tacks out of the box, fix the box to the board and put the candle in the box. You can see a video about this topic at www.bkmnutrition.com/the-candle-problem.

A great many clients come to me with the desire to lose a certain amount of weight within a set time period. I work primarily in my one-to-one practice with people who are managers or business owners and so are used to deadlines and target goals.

This is not a sensible practice for weight loss. The reason for this is that weight loss is never linear. Quite regularly I will see clients make great progress and then stall for a certain number of weeks, sometimes fluctuating around a few kilograms before then continuing with a downturn. Sometimes we have to instigate a diet break to get things going again, which results in a gain of weight for a week or so. I discuss diet breaks later in the book.

This non-linear action means that you cannot set targets for say 1 kg a week for the long term. Normally when someone starts a diet, they will lose weight very quickly and then start to level out. If you work to a set-in-stone weight target, what will happen is you will take shortcuts to make up for the plateau.

5. Thinking too much about the goal and not the process

By focussing on the goal, you will lose sight of the process and systems in place and become the first candle group, always focussing on the goals and never the systems. What this leads to is overly restrictive diets and excessive cardio in order to try to force the weight loss to happen within a constrained time period. This puts extra stress onto your mind and body, and actually the reverse can happen as your body fights the increase in the deficit by an adaptation to your metabolic rate and a drop in NEAT activity. Now you're really up the creek without a paddle as you have nowhere to go and you're afraid of reducing activity in case you gain weight.

Unless you are a competitive athlete who needs to make weight then you should never apply a time constraint to your weight-loss goals. I go even further with clients and we don't set weight-loss goals either.

Hold on, no weight-loss goals? What kind of fat-loss coach are you? I'm actually not a fat-loss coach, I am a leaner lifestyle coach. Fat loss is something that happens from living a leaner lifestyle. The goal is the lifestyle, the things that happen as a result are fat loss, greater health and more energy for life.

Imagine that you set yourself a target of losing 20 kg and that was where you think you'd be happy with your body shape. You achieve that goal, but you still have visible fat to lose. Would you think you'd succeeded or failed?

Now imagine that you set yourself a goal of 20 kg and you lost 19 kg and look great, but whatever you do you can't reach 20 kg. Would you have succeeded or failed?

Both these situations are measured by one key variable – the 20 kg of weight. Achieving or not achieving the goal can be failure in some respect.

Now imagine this:

You start living a leaner lifestyle, you eat well, you exercise a bit more, you start to fit into clothes better and people start noticing that you are thinner. You enjoy the fact that you can eat foods that you like and still lose weight, there's no time constraint as you're happy to see the results come in as you are pursuing this new leaner identity and all the benefits it brings in addition to the fat loss.

- You lose 19 kg; you look fantastic and you are happy with how you look, and you can maintain it through your new lifestyle. You've succeeded
- You lose 20 kg; you're happy with your progress but there's more to come off and you are confident you can continue the progress by following the systems and processes that you've laid out

By removing the weight goal and the time constraint you've removed the urgency and the temporary nature of the change. You are not trying to lose weight; you are living like a leaner person.

Do you still want to focus on the weight-loss goal?

71. DIET BREAKS

This entire book has been focussed on the diet. Let's take a break for a moment to think about diet breaks and eating more food to lose weight.

"Now you're talking," I hear you cry, *"bring on the cake and ice cream."*

Well, yes and no. Diet breaks are a planned mission that involves an increase in food at key points of the diet. However, it's not a licence to 'kill the buffet', 007. The premise of this method is as follows: when you have been dieting for a while your body compensates for the reduction in intake by slightly reducing your metabolic rate and increasing your hunger. The key hormones responsible for this are thyroid, leptin and ghrelin, amongst others. This is not a science-heavy book, so I won't be going into huge detail but for the purpose of this discussion these hormones start to slow down your activity during the day so that your output becomes lower and you become lazier. At the same time, you start to have more cravings for calorie-dense food and your hunger generally is more pronounced.

This means that you are more susceptible to emergences of your Muncher brain under stress situations, and even with all the coping mechanisms that I've outlined earlier, you are more likely to crack eventually.

In addition to this, your weight and fat loss starts to slow down and this can have a mental effect in terms of you thinking that you have to restrict even more, or do more cardio, which in itself does solve the issue temporarily but then the body adapts again and now you are more hungry and more tired.

The solution is to schedule a short-term increase in calories. This has the effect of resetting all your hunger and metabolic hormones so that they return to normal levels. Of course, this will result in a short-term weight gain from the extra food, which can be depressing for many people so it's very important that you are prepared for this and accept it as part of the process. After about three to five days of higher calories you can return to your diet and the resulting deficit, combined with the increased metabolism, will begin the weight-loss process again and you will drop below your plateau weight. Think of it as taking one step back in order to power forward three steps.

An important note here is that to get the real benefits of this process the increase in calories should be mainly from carbohydrate sources and not fat. Carbs generally have a better effect on thyroid and leptin levels, and in my experience working with clients the higher-carb approach tends to give the shortest duration of weight gain and the quicker return to a weight-loss environment.

A second important note is that you must have been really following the diet before doing a diet break. It's worthless to go on a diet for a few weeks and then decide it's too tough and you need a diet break, chances are you don't need one, it's more likely your diet is too strict. By doing a diet break at this point you are likely doing more harm than good. You need to be consistently in a deficit for around eight weeks and seeing a real plateau for it to be an effective process.

Diet breaks provide a number of key benefits when done right. These involve the three Cs:

- They establish choice and your control over the diet rather than being in a prison
- You'll gain a mental strength boost and clarity of knowledge eliminating confusion
- They allow consistency of the diet to be continued and frustration at lack of progress is abolished

72. WEAPON OF CHOICE

I'm a firm believer in people deciding on their own type of diet structure to fit their lifestyle. That being said, there are a number of diet structures that I've found effective for a number of my clients and I would estimate that 90% of them fall into these models. I've included them here to give you an idea of what works in the real world.

5:2 Week

This model focusses on the weekend as the highlight of the week and it suits people who work regular Monday to Friday jobs, if that sort of thing actually exists anymore. Most of my business owner and manager clients opt for this structure, as it fits in perfectly with their working week.

The structure is that you apportion more of your average calories in the week into the two weekend days and eat less Monday to Friday. An example would be:

Standard week of the same calories:
2,500 kcal every day = 17,500 kcal per week.

5:2 Week:
5 days at 2,000 kcal,
2 days at 3,750 kcal = 17,500 kcal per week.

This structure allows more calories to eat at weekends from a meal out, ice cream, some alcohol. The average calories per day is the same over seven days and you eat the same total calories for the week. Remember that the body does not work on single days but on averages over two to four weeks for long-term changes.

Intermittent fasting

This model suits people who prefer not to eat breakfast, perfectly. There is no magic metabolic boost that breakfast provides, and the research shows that when calories are matched there's no advantage or disadvantage to eating first thing in the morning in terms of weight loss.

Some of my clients prefer not to eat first thing as they are not hungry and would rather save up their calories for the day into their lunch or evening meal. A typical day may look like this:

Standard day of 2,500 kcal:

Breakfast	–	700 kcal
Lunch	–	700 kcal
Dinner	–	700 kcal
Snacks	–	400 kcal

Intermittent fasting day of 2,500 kcal:

Breakfast	–	Black coffee, 1 kcal
Lunch	–	1,000 kcal
Dinner	–	1,000 kcal
Snacks	–	499 kcal

Although coffee is pretty much zero calories when black, I added 1 kcal to keep the zealots happy. Hi, zealots!

Again, following the total calories rule we can see that the total calories over the day are the same. It's also worth noting that you can run the intermittent fasting day model with the 5:2 weekly model and so have a super-duper feast on a Saturday night. When you see my clients posting about having a Domino's and being 'on plan' that's generally how they've done it. Amazing.

Alternate-week dieting

This one takes a little more planning and involves tracking your calories over two weeks instead of one. The idea is that you deplete yourself harder for one week and then eat slightly more the next with the average of the weeks still being in a deficit.

An example would be as follows:

Standard 2 weeks:
7 x 2,500 +7 x 2,500 = 17,500 + 17,500 = 35,000 kcal.

Alternate model:
7 x 2,000 + 7 x 3,000 = 14,000 + 21,000 = 35,000 kcal.

A recent study called the MATADOR study assessed this technique and found equal weight loss between the two groups. Again, we see that the emphasis is not on one day but on an average of a few weeks.

Clients have normally followed this approach when they know that they have busy weeks coming up where they will need more calories and don't really want to compromise their progress by going to maintenance.

This approach is useful, but it can be problematic to keep track of unless you are really good at logging your calories and planning out for two weeks.

73. FAT-LOSS SUPPLEMENTS THAT WORK

This may be possibly the shortest section in any book.

1. None that are legal
2. For obvious reasons I won't be discussing illegal drugs for fat-burning here
3. Even then, you still need a calorie deficit

Supplements that may help you when trying to lose weight

While no legal fat burners exist, there are a few supplements that may help you in improving your body composition.

1. **Krill Oil and high EPA fish oils**

   In studies involving krill oil and fish oils that are high in EPA which is an omega-3 fatty acid, the subjects taking the oils improved their body composition compared to those that didn't. There is also a very beneficial effect on cholesterol from krill oil supplementation as well as cardiac health. For this reason, I always include krill oil and fish oils in my client's advisory pack. The risk of harm is negligible, and the possible benefits are huge. One client that I was advising for bodybuilding shows who had chronically high cholesterol, partly from genetics and partly from the performance enhancing drugs he was using, dropped his cholesterol by a significant factor, so much so that his doctor asked him what he was taking.

Note

Vegans and vegetarians need to use a sea algae omega-3 source to see this benefit. Plant-based omega-3 sources are not as effective as they compete for a receptor with omega-6 fatty acids, which are normally quite high in plant-based diets.

2. L-carnitine L-tartrate

The benefits from LCLT are seen after six months, which doesn't make it a quick-fix supplement. I've used it with clients for a few years, mainly with PCOS clients, because of the benefits on insulin sensitivity and its ability to help fat to enter the cells of the body to be burned as energy. Generally, it's a supplement that I've found women benefit from more in terms of body composition, and both men and women benefit from performance improvement after around six months.

If you decide to take it then the dose used in studies was 2 g per day. Make sure that you don't take it with a protein shake or high protein meal, it should be used with carbohydrate snacks for best uptake. Protein tends to interfere with absorption. Its benefits in studies was to allow better use of fat for fuel in exercise of sub-maximal output; jogging, weight training and some contact sports may benefit from its use. It must be used continually for six months, so you need to be consistent with your supplementation.

3. Caffeine

Caffeine can have a beneficial effect on fat use for fuel by stimulating adrenaline, which can in turn affect an enzyme called hormone-sensitive lipase. A number of cascading effects happen, which results in fatty acids being released from adipose tissue. It's worth pointing out that this does not make it a 'fat burner' it's just facilitating fat being able to be released into the blood. In many cases the fat that is released will be re-esterified into adipose tissue if it is not used for fuel. Caffeine is probably more beneficial for its stimulant properties, which can in turn enhance the output of your workouts. More output in workouts means more calories burned, and if your calories stay the same in a deficit, then there's a high chance that this may mean more body fat is burned over an average period.

4. **High protein intake**

This is a weird one. There has been a good deal of research into high protein intake and its effect on body composition. The curious finding is that when you increase intake from protein, even to super high levels such as 4 g per kg of bodyweight, (that's loads), the only effect on the body is to improve body composition. In simple terms, if you eat high protein you tend to be leaner than other people if other conditions are matched.

The exact mechanism for this is not known, it is the subject of much debate at the time of writing. However, for our purposes and your diet plan, I'd suggest keeping protein at a higher level to hedge your bets. Protein tends to be more satiating as a nutrient and can keep you fuller for longer and so helps greatly with dieting when hunger can be an issue.

Guideline protein amounts

I typically aim for between 1.8–2.5 g of protein per kg of bodyweight with clients. This is the level that has been agreed on by a number of researchers in the area of sports nutrition as optimal for muscle gain. For a 100 kg man this would be between 180 g–250 g per day. If you are a woman looking to lose body fat, I'd suggest aiming for between 1.8–2.0 g, as unfortunately women tend to have fewer calories to play with on a fat-loss diet.

> From a purely anecdotal perspective, I've run higher than 2.0 g per kg bodyweight protein diets with females who have hit a sticking point and seen improvements in body composition. We changed no other variables and actually increased overall calorie intake by adding in extra protein and they became leaner as a result, so it's worth considering if you have hit a sticking point and are unsure what to do.

There are many other fat-loss supplements on the market and my advice would be to treat with much scepticism. Things that work *really* well also tend to be banned drugs or strong stimulants. Stimulants can give you a similar effect to caffeine, or stronger, but also tend to give you a huge comedown afterwards.

I've listed the ones that I use with clients and as you can see it's not a huge list. This book may, of course, be out of date in terms of research as soon as it's printed, so I would recommend always checking supplements with www.examine.com – it's a site devoted to the research of supplements and their claims and is completely self-funded to remove any bias towards companies that sell supplements. This is where I check most of my data as they also list the research studies used in their articles.

Things I *definitely* wouldn't bother with for fat loss:

- CLA
- Green tea
- Any *detox* products

- Raspberry ketones.
- HMB – an amino acid
- BHB – ketone salts
- Fasted Cardio – no better on balance than normal cardio
- Gluten-free stuff
- Anything that says it's as strong as a drug – it's not
- Anything with these words – boost, incinerate, burn, metabolism, dissolve, melt
- Anything 'proven in research/science' – probably a lie or a huge exaggeration

Not an exhaustive list but hopefully you get the idea.

74. OVER TO YOU

I grew up in the 80s, a time before the internet or smart phones. If I wanted to see my mates, I had to call them on the landline from my house. I have three other siblings, which made our family six strong. One of our traditions was to do huge jigsaw puzzles on our living room table. These were 1,000 pieces in number and took an absolute age to complete. With no social media to distract us, we would quite regularly sit for hours solving the puzzles together.

When facing the prospect of losing weight, it can sometimes feel like one of those annoying jigsaws that's a picture of a million baked beans or a brick wall. You know that there is a solution, and that others have done it, but it seems impossible even knowing where to start.

This book has given you a step-by-step guide to solving your own puzzle. When solving jigsaws, it's best to collect all the edges first and piece them all together so that you work inwards. With diets you start with the calories and work onwards.

I absolutely believe that you will succeed in your fat-loss goals if you take on board the principles and techniques outlined here. I've been coaching clients on the Target Lean programme since 2016, and the people that get the most out of the programme are the ones that follow the C.A.L.O.R.I.E. system. They put the work in at the beginning so that they build a bridge over their previous failures. Every now and again they have a wobble and gain some weight back, but because they have laid that foundation, they easily get on the right track again.

All my clients are looking to improve on their successes in some way. I've never met anyone who is 100% happy with how they look. I think it's a good thing to want to improve or you get complacent and start to go backwards. The most important thing that I hope you get from this book is that you absolutely do not have to accept that you'll always have those fatty hips, dad bod, bingo wings or love handles.

I want you to take all the principles in this book, apply them to your life, build some powerful habits and feel confident walking on a beach again. I want you to go out clothes shopping and buy the things you want and not the ones that are only made in the bigger sizes. I want you to look in the mirror and feel sexy and attractive, then pounce on your partner without banging your head or knees because the light is off.

These are all the things that previous Target Lean members have listed as their successes. No one really ever sets out to lose weight, there's always that '*why?*' behind any diet. What's your *why*? Find it, hold on to it in your mind and never lose sight of it.

You have the power to change your body. All the tools that you need are contained in these pages. How you wield those tools will determine your eventual success.

But never, *ever* let anyone convince you that you are stuck with how you look forever. Take control of your life, follow the C.A.L.O.R.I.E. system and go get some shit done to look incredible.

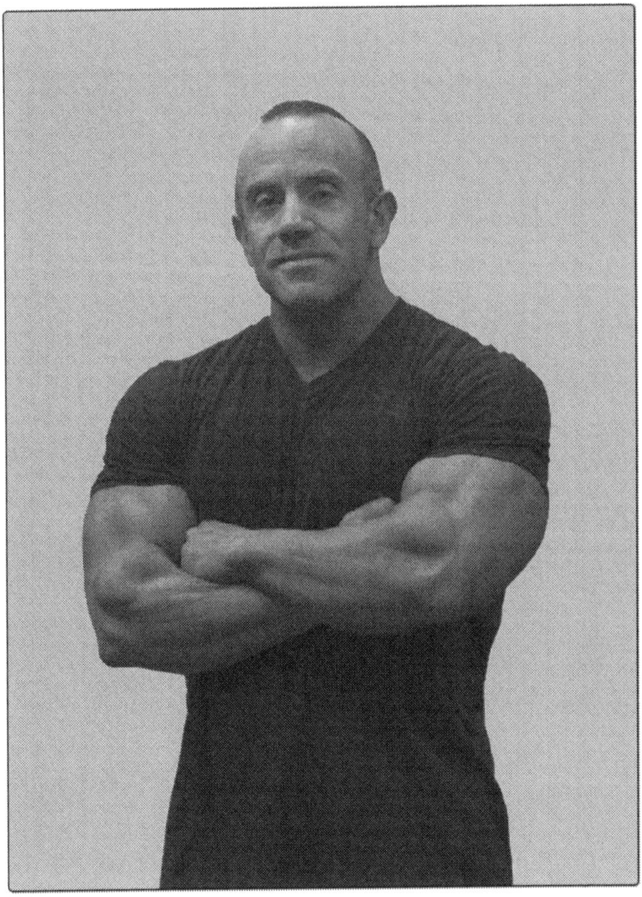

ABOUT THE AUTHOR

Tom Blackman is a performance nutritionist who graduated with distinction in Applied Sports and Exercise Nutrition from the International Society of Sports Nutrition. He is a former champion bodybuilder with over 10 years competitive experience. After retiring from competition in 2015 and recording 6 months of his life for a documentary called 'Prep the series', which was watched in over 40 countries worldwide, he turned his career to nutrition.

Initially working with champion athletes, both amateur and professional, in Mixed Martial Arts, Powerlifting, Bodybuilding and Boxing he moved into providing nutrition consulting for business owners, many of whom were parents. A parent himself, Tom understood the huge demands of running a business as well as having a busy family life. This allowed him to create nutrition and training programs for his clients so that they could get into incredible shape while still enjoying their family days out and improving their performance at work.

Tom regularly teaches clients how to adapt their lifestyle to 'eat happy'. Achieving the body they want while eating foods that they like. He has trademarked a process called the 'DIET Ecosystem' which determines where someone needs to improve in order to achieve the results they want. He also runs the Target Lean program which inspired the book and many of the techniques from the book are directly used with clients in his programs.

CONTACT THE AUTHOR

www.bkmnutrition.com

www.facebook.com/BKMNutrition

www.linkedin.com/in/tomblackman-nutrition/

www.instagram.com/tomblackman_nutrition/

www.youtube.com/c/TomBlackman

Printed in Great Britain
by Amazon

39988991R00156